The IMMUNOTHERAPY MIRACLE!

Victory in the War on Cancer

How Nobel Prize Winning FDA Approved "Checkpoint Inhibitors" CHECKMATE Cancer By *UNLEASHING* the IMMUNE SYSTEM'S *"WARRIORS WITHIN"* TO FIND, DESTROY, AND REMEMBER CANCER CELLS WITHOUT TOXINS!

From Stage 4 to "No Detectible Signs of Cancer!"

Written and Compiled by

NutraScience Research, LLC

LYNNE MEREDITH,

B.S., Certified Health Specialist,

Director of Research and Development

"Immunotherapy capitalizes on the innate power of the immune system to eliminate cancer, giving patients hope for a cure. By taking advantage of our immune system's ability to remember cancer cells, there is the potential to offer permanent protection against cancer's recurrence."
CRI Cancer Research Institute

The IMMUNOTHERAPY MIRACLE!
Victory in the War on Cancer!

Written and Compiled by
NutraScience Research, LLC

LYNNE MEREDITH,
B.S., Certified Health Specialist,

Director of Research and Development

Paperback: 978-1-967632-43-5

Hardcover: 978-1-967632-44-2

eBook: 978-1-967632-45-9

Printed in the United States of America

DEDICATION

This book is dedicated to every person who the hell of cancer has ever touched; to those who have died from cancer after a noble battle, as well as those who have been tormented by the loss of family, loved ones, and friends .

It is dedicated to the brilliant men and women who made the life-saving discoveries on how to harness the immune system to destroy cancer cells, and who were VICTORIOUS in the War on Cancer, and to the Creator of our magnificent immune system and the "Healers Within."

It is dedicated to my maternal grandmother, who died of breast cancer, and was taken from me and my brothers when I was eight years old, and she was 41. It is dedicated to my family, who supported me through my battle with cancer, including my three adult children, nine grandchildren, one great-granddaughter, and the one on the way. I pray they will grow up in a World Free From Cancer based on the pivotal discoveries incorporated in this book.

It is also dedicated to my five brothers and their wives for always creating a support system for me, and to my nieces and nephews.

It is dedicated to my mother, who was always my greatest supporter in my crusades for justice. It is also dedicated to my father, for my insatiable curiosity genes, and to my paternal grandmother, for my feisty genes.

TABLE OF CONTENTS

PART TWO

ENHANCING THE EFFICACY OF IMMUNOTHERAPY

FOREWARD

By Marianne Williamson

PHASE 1

In every generation, there are battles that define the human journey, not merely because of the physical suffering they inflict, but because of the spiritual questions they force us to confront. The war on cancer has been one such battle. It has been a saga of courage and heartbreak, of scientific exploration and soul-deep yearning for a future free from the relentless grip of cancer, a disease that has touched nearly every family, every community, every life.

The Immunotherapy Miracle! Victory in the War on Cancer is more than a chronicle of medical discovery. It is a trumpet call to our higher capacities, a celebration of the union of science and spirit, and a testament to what becomes possible when love, intelligence, and a refusal to surrender coalesce.

For decades, we have lived under the long shadow of cancer a diagnosis that has often felt like a death sentence, or at best, an invitation to a painful and uncertain path. The sheer randomness of it has haunted us. Cancer has never cared who you are, how old you are, how good you've been. It has struck down children and elders, the strong and the vulnerable, leaving behind stories too heavy for words and pain that can only be carried by the heart.

But this book tells another story. A story of hope. A story of healing. A story of victory not in the sense of dominance over nature, but in harmony with it. For what immunotherapy represents is not just a medical breakthrough; it is a reawakening of the most profound principle in healing that the body is not our enemy, but our ally. That within us lives the intelligence and power not only to endure disease, but to transcend it.

Immunotherapy, at its essence, is a scientific rediscovery of the body's own capacity to defend and restore itself. Rather than poisoning cancer cells through radiation or chemotherapy, immunotherapy teaches the body to recognize the threat, to remember it, and to remove it. It speaks not only to the brilliance of medical research, but to the deeper spiritual truth that healing is an inside-out process. The miracle, in this case, is not found in the treatment or the lab alone. It is found in awakening what has been dormant within us.

There's something profoundly spiritual about that. In every spiritual tradition, we are taught that there is a light within us, a spark of divine intelligence that can never be fully extinguished. What if this light lives not only in our consciousness, but also in our cells? What if the wisdom of the body is simply a reflection of the wisdom of the soul? In many ways, cancer has challenged us to evolve. It has exposed not just our biological vulnerabilities but our emotional, psychological, and spiritual ones as well.

The stress of modern life, the toxins in our environment, the ways in which we have often lived out of balance with nature and ourselves all these things create a terrain in which illness can thrive. But so too can health. So too can resilience. And now, with the advent of immunotherapy, we are witnessing an age in which medicine is not only more effective, but more aligned with our wholeness.

PHASE 2

This book is timely, not just because of the scientific achievements it outlines, but because of the spiritual readiness it speaks to. We are living in an era of awakening. More and more people are recognizing that health is not merely the absence of disease, but the presence of vitality, peace, and alignment with our deepest selves. Immunotherapy, in its finest expression, honors this truth. It doesn't just attack disease, it activates wellness.

But make no mistake: this is also a book about courage. The courage of the scientists who refused to accept the limitations of old paradigms. The courage of the patients who volunteered for trials, not knowing what would come. The courage of families who held onto faith when medicine had no more answers. And the courage of those who lost their lives, yet whose stories and sacrifices laid the foundation for the miracles we are now witnessing.

In these pages, you will find both data and destiny. You will read about therapies that have transformed terminal diagnoses into long-term remission.

The Immunotherapy Miracle!

You will learn about targeted treatments that bypass the toxic treatments of the past that destroy every fast growing cell in the body along with the cancer cells. But more than that, you will come to see that we are not helpless. That cancer is not an invincible enemy. That love, coupled with intelligence, is the most powerful medicine of all.

Let us not forget: healing is not only about science. Healing is about relationships, our relationship with our bodies, with our physicians, with our communities, with the Earth, and with the mystery of life itself. It is about reclaiming the narrative of illness not as a punishment, but as a call to transformation. And in that transformation, miracles are not only possible they are inevitable.

The Immunotherapy Miracle gives us more than information; it gives us vision. It asks us to imagine a world where cancer is no longer a death sentence, where the immune system is honored and empowered, where healing is approached with reverence and not just fear. It invites us to see medicine as a sacred art as much as a science.

As someone who has spent my life advocating for the politics of love and a culture of compassion, I see this book as part of that revolution.

Because true healing is never just about the individual, it ripples outward. When one person is cured, a family is restored. When one life is saved, a future is born. When one disease is defeated, a generation finds hope.

So let us celebrate this moment. Let us honor the journey. Let us remember those who have lost their lives to cancer, and cherish those we can now save. And let us move forward not just in scientific achievement, but in collective consciousness.

PHASE 3

The war on cancer has not merely been fought in labs and hospitals; it has been fought in hearts and homes, in prayers and in poems, in the quiet strength of caregivers and the fierce will of survivors. This book is their anthem. It is their vindication. It is their miracle.

And for all of us regardless of our past, our diagnosis, or our story it is a promise: that healing is possible, that the body is wise, and that when love and science walk hand in hand, even the darkest night can give way to dawn.

PHASE 4

One where the immune system, this quiet miracle within us, is being seen not as an afterthought, but as the leading character in our healing journey. One where medicine does not silence the body, but listens to it! There is something sacred in that shift.

When we begin to treat illness not as a punishment but as a signal a call to deeper listening, to greater balance, to radical self-love we change not just our health, but our consciousness. We begin to understand that healing is never just physical. It is emotional. It is spiritual. It is relational. It is, ultimately, love made manifest.

The Immunotherapy Miracle is more than a book. It is a declaration. It declares that we are stepping into a future in which medicine honors not only the body, but the spirit. It declares that our greatest breakthroughs come not from conquering nature, but from harmonizing with it. It declares that within the very cells of our being lives a holy light that can be reawakened.

PHASE 5

This is not to say the journey has been easy. It has not. It has taken decades of research, the loss of lives, the enduring grief of families, and the steadfastness of believers. But from that darkness has come something radiant. A treatment that doesn't just promise survival but restores dignity.

A hope that doesn't just comfort but delivers.

The direction is clear. The momentum is real. And the victory, while still unfolding, is no longer just a dream. It is happening.
And as with all true miracles, this one is rooted not only in science but in love. Love for life. Love for truth. Love for one another.

Let this book be your companion on this journey, whether you are a patient, a caregiver, a physician, or simply someone seeking to understand what is emerging. May it inform you, yes, but may it also inspire you. May it help you to trust again in the wisdom of your body, the goodness of others, and the potential for light to return where darkness once lived.

Marianne Williamson 🧡 100%!

ABOUT THE FORWARD AUTHOR

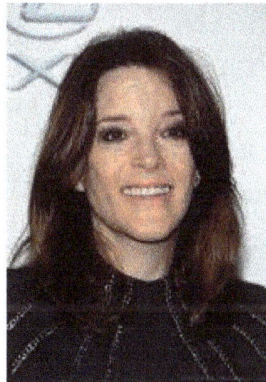

Marianne Williamson has authored sixteen books, seven of which were New York Times bestsellers. Her notable works include *A Return to Love* (1992), *An Age of Miracles*, *Every Day Grace*, *The Law of Divine Compensation*, *Illuminata*, *A Woman's Worth*, *The Healing of America*, and *The Mystic Jesus*. She gained recognition through regular appearances on Oprah Winfrey's show as her "spiritual advisor." Williamson ran for President in 2020 and 2024, advocating for a U.S. Department of Peace, and also ran for California's 33rd congressional district in 2014, placing fourth with 13.2% of the vote. Her charitable work includes founding the Center for Living (1987), Project Angel Food (1989), and the Peace Alliance (1998). She serves on the board of RESULTS, a nonprofit focused on ending poverty.

PREFACE

> **"For the first time, we can use the word 'cure' in the same sentence as cancer."** James P. Allison, PhD, Nobel Laureate

I should be dead now, but I am a living testament to the miraculousness of immunotherapy and the power of the immune system to destroy cancer.

The profound scientific discoveries contained in this book saved my life when I was diagnosed with Stage IV cancer that had spread throughout my bones, my liver, and into my skull.

I am "alive by science," and the discoveries of brilliant Cancer Research Scientists who developed immunotherapy checkpoint inhibitors, which checkmate cancer, by exposing the previously hidden immune system and unleashing the power of the immune system to find, mark, destroy, and remember cancer cells without toxins, while leaving healthy cells intact.

Knowledge is power, and knowledge that can save lives is the ultimate power.

My mission in creating this book is to create IMMUNOTHERAPY AWARENESS by sharing recent discoveries that can **END CANCER,** without chemotherapy or radiation. My goal is to make Immunotherapy common knowledge by educating the *critical mass* of people about recently discovered Immunotherapy Checkpoint Inhibitors.

This miraculous cancer treatment consists of a simple, nontoxic 30-minute infusion every three weeks.

It can unleash the body's own immune system to reverse even cancers once thought to be death sentences, such as metastatic melanoma and small cell lung cancer, as well as about 30 other types of cancer.

Immunotherapy is a Nobel Prize-winning and FDA-approved treatment that is currently recognized as the Fourth Standard of Care for cancer treatments, which previously included only surgery, chemotherapy, and radiation. This means that any oncologist or physician can prescribe immunotherapy checkpoint inhibitors without fear of losing their Medical License.

Immunotherapy is administered in the same infusion centers that provide chemotherapy or other types of infusions.

The information in this book, when shared, can also save the lives of others and end the agony and terror of cancer without toxic chemotherapy or radiation.

Immunotherapy Checkpoint Inhibitors harness the body's immune system to recognize previously hidden cancer cells, to find, destroy, flag, and remember them. It is a watershed Victory in the War on Cancer!

INTRODUCTION

Immunotherapy has significantly impacted cancer survival rates and has contributed to a significant decline in cancer deaths, saving millions of lives. A report by the American Association for Cancer Research (AACR) shows that breakthroughs in immunotherapy have contributed to a 33% decrease in cancer death rates, saving an estimated 3.8 million lives. Successful treatment has been achieved in over 30 types of cancer and counting.

For patients who respond to immunotherapy checkpoint inhibitors and show no disease progression for at least three years, there's the potential for a long-term cure.

Studies show that the benefits of immunotherapy can continue after the treatment has stopped.

Immunotherapy has revolutionized the treatment of several cancers that were once considered death sentences, significantly improving patient outcomes and offering new hope. Stage four Melanoma was virtually a death sentence, with patients surviving, on average, less than a year. Thanks to immunotherapy, particularly immune checkpoint inhibitors like pembrolizumab and nivolumab, survival rates for patients with advanced Melanoma have dramatically increased.

Non-small cell lung cancer was historically considered to be the deadliest of all cancers. However, immunotherapy has significantly changed this and has helped drive a substantial decline in lung cancer deaths.

If you have cancer, have ever had cancer, know someone who does, or if you think that you may ever get cancer, this book could save your life or the life of someone else. Immunotherapy can also take the fear out of cancer.

When you're diagnosed, there are many decisions to make, while emotions are high, and much is unknown. Having a game plan and making an "educated decision" about your treatment could mean the difference between life and death and your quality of life during treatment.

Now, in addition to choices of Surgery, Chemotherapy, and Radiation, there is Checkpoint Inhibitor Immunotherapy.

This new FDA-approved, Nobel Prize-winning treatment, recognized as the **Fourth Standard of Care.** It commandeers the "warriors within" (the body's immune system) to annihilate cancer without toxins. Immunotherapy only requires a thirty-minute painless infusion every three weeks.

Also, *mutant* p53 genes, which instruct cells to stop growing, that are prevalent in many cancers, can be targeted by immunotherapy to restore their cancer tumor suppressive function. Immunotherapy may also restore the mutant p21's function of facilitating cell cycle arrest.

CHAPTER ONE

Immunotherapy Checkpoint Inhibitor

SURVIVOR STORIES

Author Lynne Meredith's Victory Over Cancer With Immunotherapy

In May of 2023, after my oldest brother, Glen, and my sister in law, Joanne, had taken me to lunch, I complained of pain at the top junction of my leg and pubic bone as I was walking back to my car. They feared that I might have had a blood clot, which ran in our family. Knowing my propensity to procrastinate, in an act of kindness that probably saved my life, they showed up at my front door the next morning to take me to Cedars-Sinai Hospital for a CT scan.

The Scan showed I had no clots. However, it found two lesions on me at the top of my left leg. A biopsy showed that the tumors were high-grade leiomyosarcoma. The oncologist's words echoed through my ears: ***"You've got cancer,"*** stated with the same lack of emotion as "You've got mail." He explained to me that the alien that had invaded my body had a name.

It was called 'Leiomyosarcoma,' or LMS, which is a rare type of soft tissue cancer that grows rapidly in the smooth muscles of the body.

When discussing treatments, I knew that I didn't want chemotherapy or radiation.

My earliest memory of cancer was on March 1, 1958, on my 8th Birthday. My maternal grandmother phoned me, and my mom took me to visit her. It was a few days before she died, at the young age of 41, from breast cancer.

She had undergone massive chemotherapy and radiation and was a tragic, skeletal, skin and bones image of her prior, vivacious self. She had a bucket next to her. She was profusely vomiting, and her eyes looked bloody.

This terrifying image was the last time I saw the grandmother, whom I adored, alive.

I knew I didn't want chemo or radiation, so I looked for less invasive choices. I decided on "Cryoablation." It uses a CT scan to locate the tumor and then freezes it to kill it.

This turned out to be a bad choice. The freezing temperatures froze my thinning bones and cracked my pelvis, tailbone, and other bones. I had to go to a rehab for a month, where I learned to learn to walk again.

I moved to Boise to be close to my two daughters, who lived there.

I was cancer-free for approximately nine months.

The Immunotherapy Miracle!

Then another tumor grew in my lower abdomen that turned out to be another highly aggressive Leiomyosarcoma lesion.

I opted for surgery to remove it but refused chemo and radiation.

However, I also had contracted Bell's Palsy, which partially paralyzed the left side of my face, and the cancer surgeons delayed my surgery for three months, waiting for it to heal.

The abdominal tumor was finally surgically removed.

A later MRI showed that, even though the tumor in my abdomen was gone, cancer had spread through my pelvic bones, ribs, and spine, and had metastasized to my liver. I also had five cancerous lesions on my skull. I could feel a walnut-sized tumor on the right side of my skull and could not hear out of my right ear. The pain in my bones and liver was excruciating. I couldn't roll over in bed or walk without pain. I needed a wheelchair to get around.

I no longer felt like myself. I felt like I was dying, and the oncologist had concurred. I was passionate about life, my family, and my friends. I had three adult children (Kari, Erik, and Jeni). I was also the proud "Nana" of nine grandchildren. Additionally. I had four younger brothers whom I adored. I wasn't ready to leave this planet. Like the Kenny Chesney song says, "Everybody wants to go to Heaven, but nobody wanna go NOW." I felt the most devastating sadness I had ever felt in my life.

Because the cancer had spread throughout my entire body, I felt that my **only** hope for survival was **immunotherapy**.

During my cancer ordeal, I had asked three oncologists how to obtain it, but was always referred back to systemic chemotherapy and radiation, which I had no interest in. They would have only prolonged my suffering.

I started advocating for myself because my life depended upon it.

I hold a BS degree with a focus in Nutritional Science and serve as the Director of Research and Development for NutraScience Research. LLC. I made a crucial "executive decision" to make "Immunotherapy Checkpoint Inhibitors" an immediate, extensive research project. I also wanted to help others suffering from cancer. We've lost too many people to the disease.

I decided I wanted an "Immunotherapy checkpoint inhibitor," called pembrolizumab (Keytruda). Even though it had not been approved for my type of cancer, I hoped that because our immune system patrols our entire body, it would still find and destroy the cancer. It was my only hope.

I started by researching how to obtain it. First, I called my Health Insurance to see if they covered it. I was informed that it was not on their list of approved medications. However, the insurance person was kind enough to explain that they could cover it if my oncologist said that ***"It was medically necessary."***

I then went directly to the source and called the manufacturer Merck at (855) 398-7832. They were extremely *"customer centric."* The person I talked to was very kind and helpful. She gave me the following website for the

Merck Access Program: www.merckaccessportal.com

There, I found the following information: "Merck provides certain types of its medicines for free to eligible patients who do not have prescription drug or health insurance coverage and who, without assistance, cannot afford the medicines and vaccines made by Merck. This is consistent with Merck's long-held values and tradition of putting patients first.

If you need further information or help paying for KEYTRUDA, Merck may be able to help. Contact the Merck Access Program at 855-257-3932."

From there, I enrolled at:

www.merckaccessprogram-keytruda.com

Merck emailed me a Form. I downloaded it, filled out my part, and took it to the Oncologist's office.

I gave the Form to the person in charge of collecting medical payments, and she had the rest of the Form filled out and signed by my Oncologist and faxed it back to: 855-755-0518. It can also be submitted electronically.

Within two weeks, I started my first 30-minute infusion of Keytruda (Pembrolizumab)! I was ELATED and felt I had a second chance at life!

I chose pembrolizumab (Ketruda), but a patient could go through the same process with other checkpoint inhibitors. The oncologist can prescribe it. The Social Worker at the hospital can also usually help with the steps to get immunotherapy and funding for it.

The painless immunotherapy infusions took 30 minutes, every 3 weeks. They even provided lunch!

The only side effects I experienced occurred after my first infusion. I had no side effects during subsequent treatments. After the first treatment, I experienced achy bones, weak and painful muscles, and itchiness for about a week. This was because, as cancer cells are destroyed, they trigger the immune system's mast cells to release histamines. This is a good sign. However, since I have allergies, these side effects were more intense. I later discovered that the histamine-related side effects could have been avoided or diminished by taking an H-1 antihistamine (such as Allegra) before my treatments.

The oncologist suggested a long series of radiation treatments, in addition to the immunotherapy. I told him I believed the immunotherapy alone would destroy tumors without radiation or chemotherapy.

I remember a nurse telling my daughter that she should convince me to take the radiation because, otherwise, the tumors might grow out of my skull and frighten my grandchildren. Talk about a hard sell!

Lynne's Immunotherapy Miracle!

After my third infusion, the miracles began to happen!

The walnut-sized tumor on the right side of my skull, which I could feel with my hand, disappeared, and my hearing came back!

I rolled over in my bed, stood up, and started laughing as I walked without pain! I said, "Alexa, play my music," and started to dance!

I no longer needed pain pills or a wheelchair!   I was elated and cried happy tears!

I thanked God for the brilliant research scientists who learned how to unleash the immune system against cancer. They saved my life!

I walked into my third appointment and took a seat. The oncologist came in and asked, "Where's your wheelchair!?" It even surprised him.

My First Scan: All Cancerous Lesions had Disappeared or Had Dramatically Shrunk in Size!

A CT scan and MRI after nine weeks showed that all the tumors, including the bones and skull, had either completely disappeared or had dramatically shrunk. The liver tumor had shrunk by 80%!

There were no new tumors or lesions, and no new metastasis.

The immune system has "memory" to alleviate the fear it will return.

Ex President Jimmy Carter's Survival Story

"Our Immune System is the Greatest Weapon we have in our Fight Against Cancer!" Cancer Research Institute

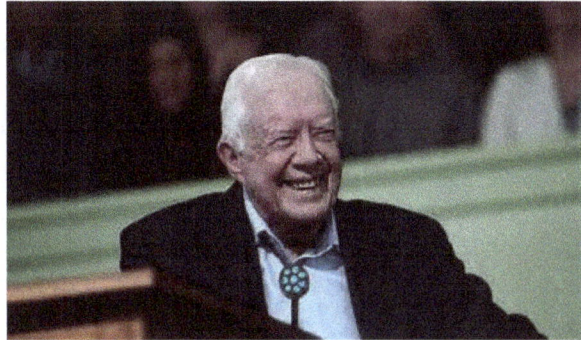

Paul Hennessy/NurPhoto via Getty

Jimmy Carter, the 39th President of the United States, was a Champion of Human Rights.

He was the face, hands, and heart of "Habitat for Humanity," which created affordable housing for those in need. He and his wife, Rosalynn, helped build, renovate, and repair over 4000 homes.

 In August of 2015, Carter was diagnosed with advanced metastatic melanoma, which at that time was considered a death sentence. The survival rate was extremely low. Most patients lived only for months or weeks.

It had also spread to his liver and four areas of his brain.

The Immunotherapy Miracle!

Carter also received radiation for his brain tumors. Medically, this can provide relief from symptoms, but it does not stop disease progression.

Carter's father, his only brother, and both sisters died of pancreatic Cancer.

Carter began the immunotherapy checkpoint inhibitor, Keytruda, in August of 2015. In December, **three months later**, his doctors announced the then-91-year-old was completely cancer-free. Scans showed that **his tumors were completely gone**. His ongoing follow-ups, starting in February 2016, showed no recurrences. Carter's images showed he was free of all cancer.

Jimmy Carter's decision to publicly discuss his Immunology treatment provided hope for thousands of people with cancer.

Carter raised awareness of Immunotherapy and opened the eyes of many doctors, patients, families, and caregivers. Numerous cancer patients simply told their oncologists, "I want what Jimmy Carter had!"

Keytruda was approved by the FDA in 2014 and by 2024 had received its 40th FDA approval for a multitude of cancers.

On May 23, 2017, pembrolizumab (Keytruda) became the first cancer treatment (of any type) to be approved by the FDA without any organ-specific strings attached.

"Cancer's Penicillin Moment: Drugs that UNLEASH The Immune System to Destroy Cancer Cells
By Andy Coghlan

"WHEN Vicky Brown was diagnosed with advanced malignant melanoma in 2013, she was in shock. Most people with even the best treatment at the time of their diagnosis lived for about six months. Then her fate took a turn for the better. Brown was referred to take part in a trial of an experimental treatment.

Over several weeks, she received three intravenous infusions.

After the second, the lumps she had felt in her throat and breast had vanished. 'I was thrilled,' says Brown, who is still alive almost three years after her initial diagnosis. The consultant says he'd never seen a result like that so quickly. Brown's results may be extraordinary, but they aren't unique.

Other people who have taken part in similar trials are still alive a decade later, despite starting with similarly bleak prognoses. This new generation of anticancer drugs – called checkpoint inhibitors – is having a profound impact! 'Melanoma and lung cancer used to be death sentences, but they're not anymore,' says Gordon Freeman at the Dana-Farber Cancer Institute. '**It's a revolution.**'"

Stage IV Melanoma Survivor:
Immunotherapy Gave Me My Life Back

Source: MD Anderson Website

Medically Reviewed | Last reviewed by an MD Anderson Cancer Center medical professional on June 12, 2019

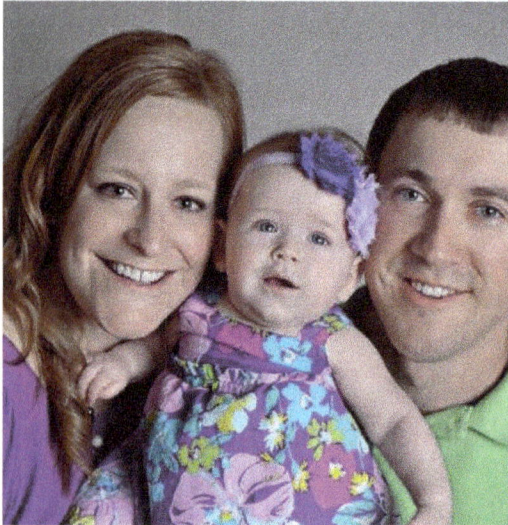

"I was diagnosed with stage IV melanoma in December 2014, a year after I had a cancerous mole removed from my left calf. I thought I was done with it.

Then I felt a lump in my groin while shaving my legs when I was 20 weeks pregnant with my second child. A lymph node biopsy revealed the melanoma was back, but it appeared to be confined to that one area. Not wanting to hurt the baby, I deferred any additional scans or treatment until after I delivered. A PET scan taken the day my son was born showed the cancer was also in my liver, spine, and other places. When I heard the results, my daughter was two, and my newborn was a week old.

I went to one of the larger hospital systems for treatment, but the chemotherapy they recommended didn't work.

All my tumors were still growing.

The doctors there told me to make the most of the time I had left. But having such a young family, I couldn't accept that prognosis.

Instead, I found a clinical trial at MD Anderson that combined two different immunotherapy drugs. It saved my life.

Why I chose a clinical trial for my melanoma treatment

I knew I was in the right place at MD Anderson when I first met with my oncologist, Dr. Isabella Glitza. She started my appointment simply listening. Then, she sketched out a list of all my options and explained each one, as well as its risks and benefits. My husband and I picked the one we thought was best: a clinical trial yielding tremendous results for people with my exact type of cancer. Fortunately, I qualified to participate, so I enrolled in the clinical trial in March 2015. But I only made it through three of my four scheduled IV infusions of ipilimumab and nivolumab.

My doctors thought the diarrhea I developed might be colitis, a known side effect of those drugs, so they took me off the trial. I was devastated. I thought for sure I hadn't received enough of the drugs to make a difference.

However, my first scans in May 2015 showed a 95% reduction in my tumors. **And by November 2015, I showed no evidence of disease at all.**

Cherishing the Time I Thought I'd Never Get

I'm not sure I can adequately express my reaction to finding out my cancer was gone. It's hard to explain how grateful I feel just to be alive. I fell asleep smiling that night.

I didn't go into the clinical trial hoping for a cure. I thought if I could just stretch out my time with my husband and children a little, that would be enough. So, I was told I was essentially cancer-free, and I couldn't believe it. It wasn't even a possibility that had crossed my mind.

Since then, I've finished grad school, celebrated birthdays and holidays, and watched both of my kids perform in plays and gymnastics. Those are all things I never thought I'd have a chance to do. So, the last four years have been amazing.

I've since learned that Nobel Prize winner, MD Anderson immunotherapy researcher, Dr. Jim Allison, is responsible (at least in part) for my survival. It was his research that led to the development of *ipilimumab*.

I like Dr. Allison's story because he seems like such a normal guy. Sometimes, I look around my small-town classroom and think, "Could one of you be the next Dr. Allison?" I've started sharing his story with my students. I think it's one that young people can learn from: it's about not giving up and believing in yourself. Dr. Allison saved many lives — including mine.

Stage IV Melanoma Survivor: An immunotherapy Drug Gave me my life back – By Mark Zindler

In early 2019, I was almost seven years out of my melanoma diagnosis.

I'd been living cancer-free since having surgery and radiation therapy during the spring of 2012. I was looking forward to retirement with my wife.

Then, during a regular follow-up visit at MD Anderson, I got a crushing blow: the cancer had returned. Scans revealed I had three new tumors. Two were in my right lung. But the third was growing in the left ventricle of my heart.

A biopsy showed that the tumors in my lungs were melanoma. So, it was logical to assume the third one was, as well. But it was too dangerous to biopsy the tumor in my heart, so I reviewed my options with my oncologist, Dr Rodale Amaria. She recommended an immunotherapy drug called *nivolumab*. I took her advice and started getting infusions of it. Within 10 months, I was cancer-free.

Hope Despite a Stage IV Diagnosis

When I first found out my cancer had returned, I thought I'd make it through the summer, maybe. The cancer was already in stage IV now, and it had invaded my heart. Cancer doesn't play fair. But Dr. Amaria gave me hope.

The drug she recommended was built for treating melanoma. And immunotherapy gives you an army of T cells to do it.

I started taking *nivolumab* in January 2019. By July, my scans showed the tumors were visibly shrinking. And by last November, my doctors could find ***no evidence of disease.*** I was blown away.

Immunotherapy made me one of the lucky ones.

I still get infusions of *nivolumab*. I'm on my 23rd dose right now. But I've been doing so well on it that Dr. Amaria says she'll be taking me off the medication in October, three months earlier than originally planned.

I've hardly had any side effects either -- just some fatigue and a rash on my back for a couple of weeks. I consider this a miracle. Because even after being diagnosed with stage IV cancer, here I am again, almost two years later, cancer-free. And I feel great.

Dr. William Lee, Author of "Eat to Beat Disease."

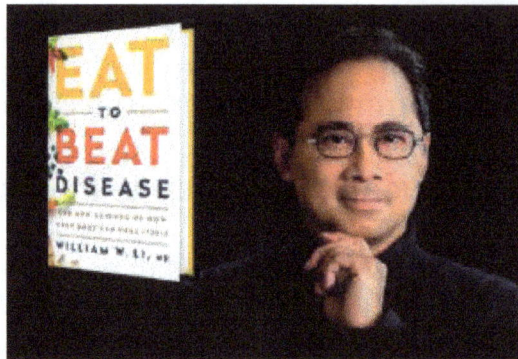

Go to the Video Link below to hear Dr. William Li, a Physician Scientist and author of EAT TO BEAT CANCER, discuss his mom's cure from multiple Stage 4, metastatic Cancers with Immunotherapy:

https://www.facebook.com/reel/1142405294044619

American Lung Association

by Editorial Staff | June 27, 2023

"Originally diagnosed with uterine cancer, Irisaida was dismayed when, after 11 months of remission, her doctors informed her that the cancer had metastasized to her lungs. She was now considered a Stage IV cancer patient and was advised to receive a lobectomy (removal of a section of the lung), followed by a standard course of chemotherapy.

After completing 6.5 hours of chemo, it became obvious that something else needed to be done. Despite the aggressive treatment, cancer had continued to spread and was now attacking the upper lobe, the pleura, and the mediastinum, completely compromising Irisaida's ability to breathe. "That is when I started seeking other options," she said.

Irisaida consulted other doctors, and it was agreed upon that she would qualify for an immunotherapy trial.

Immunotherapy works by boosting a patient's overall immune response so that it can strengthen the body and combat cancer cells.

Six months into the treatment, her cancer began to shrink, and now, two years later, there is **'no evidence of disease.'**

The number of deaths was high before options like immunotherapy. Stage IV cancer is no longer a death sentence."

From Caregiver to Cancer Survivor of Brain Cancer and Melanoma

"Jane explained how she is a living miracle, having survived and endured four major surgeries, radiation, and cancer treatments since October 2014. 'We are so blessed with medical technology right now, with **immunotherapy** and many new medications being approved every day!'

She also referred to her OHA oncologists, Dr. Roger Holden and Dr. William Cunningham, as 'a blessing' for the care and treatment they both provided. Roger Holden, MD, PhD, said, 'With extensive disease, brain cancer, and melanoma, if it were eight years ago, she wouldn't be here with us today.'

With excitement in his voice, Dr. Holden continued, 'Jane is now cancer-free',

Jun 18, 2018 #PatientStories Cancer Research Institute

K.C. Dill and Stage 3 Lung Cancer in 2015.

After receiving chemotherapy and radiation, her healthcare team was not optimistic—her cancer had spread to her lymph nodes and progressed to stage 4. K.C. sought a second opinion in Houston and began treatment with nivolumab. She responded to the immunotherapy immediately, and her recent scans show no evidence of disease. To hear her story, go to the following Link:

https://www.youtube.com/watch?v=ag4g8zlWsMo

Sixteen Plus Years Cancer Free

Thanks to Immunotherapy - Sharon Belvin - Melanoma

Sharon Belvin was one of the first patients in the world treated with an immune checkpoint inhibitor--and remains cancer-free today.

In 2004, at only 22 years old, Sharon Belvin was diagnosed with stage 4 melanoma. Running out of options, her oncologist, Dr. Jedd Wolchok of Memorial Sloan, prescribed Immunotherapy,

She shares her story to empower other cancer patients at the following website:

https://www.youtube.com/watch?v=GOr1sDQdeYw

Arlene Chivil – Getting Life Back
After Hodgkin's Lymphoma

Diagnosed with Hodgkin lymphoma while in college, Ariella Chivil completed standard treatment for the disease and hoped to put it behind her. Unfortunately, the cancer returned. After trying 14 different cancer treatments, Ariella enrolled in an **immunotherapy** clinical trial for the drug nivolumab (Opdivo). Watch her share her story at the following Link:

https://video.search.yahoo.com/search/video?fr=mcafee&p=immunotherapy+success+story&type=E211US1274G0#id=92&vid=55719184acd363ad236fb45f460f2539&action=view

I Wanted Immunotherapy!

Source: Let's Win Pancreatic Cancer www.letswinpc.org
February 6, 2024, Type of Cancer: Stage IV Pancreatic adenocarcinoma

By Daniel Miller

"In early January 2023, I began experiencing some unusual symptoms like stomach bloating, mild pain in my abdomen, and hunger pains. I was losing weight, and I always felt weak. That's when I ended up in the emergency room.

Testing and Diagnosis showed swollen lymph nodes around my aorta and stomach. That led the doctors to schedule me for more tests, including an MRI, a PET scan, a biopsy of my lymph nodes, a colonoscopy, and an endoscopy. After all those tests, I have ultimately been diagnosed with stage IV pancreatic adenocarcinoma.

Treatment

I did some research about pancreatic cancer, and from the very beginning, I knew I didn't want chemotherapy, I wanted immunotherapy!

My oncologist, Dr. Praveen Vashist at Pardee Cancer Center Hematology and Medical Oncology, part of UNC Health, in Hendersonville, North Carolina, did genetic testing and said that I could,

Dr. Vashist prescribed pembrolizumab (Keytruda) infusion at three-week intervals. It is given by infusion into a vein.

Overall, the side effects of my treatment have been minimal. I had a rash, some itching on my skin, and loose stools every now and then. I have to take ZENPEP pancreatic enzyme capsules after meals to help my digestive system work better.

Life Now

I had my 17th infusion at the end of January, along with a CT scan and blood tests. The scan shows that everything is getting smaller, and my CA 19-9 number has **dropped from over 2,000 when I was diagnosed to a number in the normal range**. I am grateful that I ended up with a positive outcome. I am Dr. Vashist's first pancreatic cancer patient.

The following is a recent excerpt related to European Clinical Studies:
15 Sep 2024 – ESMO – European Society for Medical Oncology

Lugano, Switzerland – "Immunotherapy, which works by enabling the body's immune system to recognize and destroy cancer cells, improves long-term overall survival in patients with advanced melanoma, according to results from large international studies reported at ESMO 2024. Researchers leading the longest follow-up study to date suggest that immunotherapy offers the potential for a cure in patients who respond to this treatment…

After follow-up of at least 10 years…in the CheckMate 067 trial, very few of the patients showing good initial response to anti-PD-1-based immunotherapy, with no disease progression for at least 3 years, had died of melanoma at 10 years (10-year melanoma-specific survival rate 96%).

The researchers suggested that there is now **a potential for a cure** in patients responsive to these treatments. 'The results from this trial confirm the potential for cure with immunotherapy in patients with advanced melanoma,' agreed Dr. Marco Donia, associate professor of clinical oncology at the National Center for Cancer Immune Therapy of Denmark."

CHAPTER TWO

Advantages of Immunotherapy

"Immunotherapy capitalizes on the innate power of the immune system to eliminate cancer, giving patients hope for a cure. By taking advantage of our immune system's ability to remember cancer cells, there is the potential to offer permanent protection against cancer's recurrence.
CRI Cancer Research Institute

The Miraculous New Answer to the End of Cancer!

Checkpoint Inhibitors "CHECKMATE" the Ability

of Cancer Cells to Turn Off the Immune System

According to the Cancer Research Institute, Immunotherapy "is the Smart way to fight cancer."

It's Precise

The immune system is precise, so it is possible for it to target cancer cells exclusively while sparing healthy cells.

It's Dynamic

The immune system can adapt continuously and dynamically, just like cancer does, so if a tumor manages to escape detection, the immune system can re-evaluate and launch a new attack.

It's Durable. It Remembers

The immune system's "memory" allows it to remember what cancer cells look like, so it can target and eliminate the cancer if it returns. The results may be maintained even after treatment is completed.

Previously, Chemotherapy, Surgery, and Radiation, with their hellacious side effects, were the only three *'Standards of Care'* for Cancer treatment.

Now there is a new ***Fourth*** Standard of Care, Nobel Prize-winning and FDA-approved, *Immunotherapy, Checkpoint Inhibitors*, which uses the body's immune system to locate, mark, destroy, and remember cancer cells.

The body's immune system, when working properly, is capable of eliminating cancer cells and remembering them for future destruction, **IF** it can find them. However, cancer cells have developed a unique method of turning off the immune system and *masking* themselves from T cells and the immune system, thereby evading destruction.

Astonishingly, Nobel Prize-winning and other brilliant Research Scientists, featured in this book, have discovered how to turn the immune system back on and unleash its power against cancer cells!

Immunotherapy checkpoint inhibitors require only a painless 30-minute IV infusion every three weeks, which has either no or minimal side effects; Rare, more serious side effects can typically be treated with corticosteroids.

Cancer has been found to respond incredibly well to immunotherapy treatment with immune checkpoint inhibitors, even in cancers that were previously considered death sentences.

These cancers have been shown on CT, MRI, and PET scans to go from Stage IV to "no detectible cancer."

Studies have shown Immunotherapy Checkpoint Inhibitors to be miraculously effective in treating over 30 types of cancer, including metastatic melanoma, small cell lung cancer, breast cancer, bladder cancer, cervical cancer, pancreatic cancer, colorectal cancer, kidney cancer, ovarian cancer, lung cancer, head and neck cancer, stomach, rectal cancers, and more.

According to the Cancer Research Institute, over nine million people worldwide have benefited from Immunotherapy Checkpoint Inhibitors.

Because a properly functioning immune system patrols the entire body to find, flag, destroy, and remember abnormal cancer cells, the list of cancers it can eliminate is extensive. Because of the complexity of the Immune System, Immune checkpoint inhibitor therapy has demonstrated a unique ability to treat highly malignant forms of cancer that were previously untreatable.

Check Point Inhibitor Immunotherapy has the following advantages:

Specificity

Immunotherapy is nontoxic and targets constantly mutating cancer cells, while sparing healthy cells. You won't lose your hair! It enhances your immune system for the specific purpose of killing cancer cells. Chemotherapy, discovered in 1942, has its roots in mustard gas, a chemical Weapon of War.

All types of Chemotherapy are poisonous to all fast-growing cells in the body, such as hair follicle cells and stomach cells, leading to hair loss and extreme nausea and vomiting. Chemo also attacks the bone marrow, damaging the immune system by reducing the body's white blood cells.

Immunotherapy Targets and Destroys Cancer *Stem Cell*s

Source: Targeted immunotherapy to cancer stem cells: A novel strategy of anticancer immunotherapy AShan-Yong Yi [1], Mei-Zhuo Wei [1], Ling Zhao Critical Reviews in Oncology/Hematology Volume 196, April 2024, 104313

"Since Cancer stem Cells are resistant to traditional anti-tumor therapies, researchers are turning to immunotherapeutic strategies that target Cancer Stem cells and are supported by recent preclinical studies demonstrating the effectiveness of immunotherapies in targeting Cancer Stem Cells (Chivu-Economescu et al., 2020; Codd et al., 2018; Donini et al., 2021)."

Chemotherapy Does Not Kill Cancer STEM CELLS
Which can metastasize to Another Area of the Body

Stem Cells are like seeds, which can "self renew" and can make more cells like themselves. They can also differentiate into new types of cells.

A significant disadvantage of **chemotherapy is that it does not kill cancer *stem cells***, which **evade chemotherapy**. This can cause cancer to return or metastasize to another part of the body, even after the primary tumor has been destroyed.

The following is from Yale Medicine Magazine, 2013 – Spring,

"Killing Cancer's Seeds." Anyone considering chemo should read this:

"Hope crushed can be a terrible thing. Oncologist Alessandro D. Santin, M.D., from the Yale School of Medicine, sees that despair all too often.

Most of these women undergo surgery first, then chemotherapy. After they have endured these complicated and painful treatments, often the most the doctor can offer is a small measure of good news. After chemotherapy and radiation, most patients have no detectable disease left in their bodies.

However, cancer **will return in nearly 90 percent of the apparently "cured" chemotherapy patients**—the second time *with a vengeance —and chemotherapy will no longer work.*"

Conversely, "Pre-clinical evidence suggests that immunotherapy can kill cancer stem cells in solid tumors, leading to long-term survival of the cancer patients." Source: Immune to Cancer: CRI, Cancerresearch.org

Immunotherapy has Immunological Memory

Immunotherapy Checkpoint Inhibitors harness the body's **adaptive immune system**, with Immunological Memory that allows it to remember and respond to cancer cells after treatment has ended, offering patients protection against cancer recurrence. "Immunotherapy is a 'living drug' that remains active thanks to the immune system's 'memory." CRI

CHAPTER THREE

Nobel Prize Awarded for Immunotherapy Checkpoint Inhibitors

Press release - 2018-10-01

The Nobel Assembly at Karolinska Institute awarded the 2018 Nobel Prize in Physiology or Medicine to James P. Allison and Tasuku Honjo for their discovery of cancer therapy by inhibition of negative immune regulation.

SUMMARY

"During the 1990s, in his laboratory at the University of California, Berkeley, James P. Allison studied the T-cell protein CTLA-4. He was one of several scientists who had observed that CTLA-4 functions as a brake on T cells.

…He had already developed an antibody that could bind to CTLA-4 and block its function...He now set out to investigate if CTLA-4 blockade could disengage the T-cell brake and unleash the immune system to attack cancer cells. Allison and co-workers performed their first experiment at the end of 1994, and in their excitement, it was immediately repeated over the Christmas break. The results were spectacular. Mice with cancer had been cured by treatment with the antibodies that inhibit the brake and unlock antitumor T-cell activity…

Allison continued his intense efforts to develop the strategy into a therapy for humans. Promising results soon emerged from several groups, and in 2010, an important clinical study showed striking effects in patients with advanced melanoma. In several patients, signs of remaining cancer disappeared. Such remarkable results had never been seen before in this patient group."

The Immunotherapy Miracle!

"For the first time, we can use the word 'cure' in the same sentence as cancer." James P. Allison, PhD, Nobel Laureate

In 1992, a few years before Allison's discovery, Tasuku Honjo discovered PD-1, another protein expressed on the surface of T-cells.

However, PD-1's physiologic function remained elusive for many years.

Determined to unravel its role, Honjo meticulously explored its function in a series of elegant experiments performed over many years in his laboratory at Kyoto University. The results showed that PD-1, similar to CTLA-4, functions as a T-cell brake, but operates by a different mechanism. In animal experiments, a PD-1 blockade was also shown to be a promising strategy in the fight against cancer, as demonstrated by Honjo and other groups. This paved the way for utilizing PD-1 as a target in the treatment of patients. Clinical development ensued, and in 2012, a key study demonstrated clear efficacy in the treatment of patients with different types of cancer. Results were dramatic, leading to long-term remission and possible cures in several patients with metastatic cancer, a condition that had previously been considered essentially untreatable.

After the initial studies showing the effects of CTLA-4 and \

PD-1 blockade, the clinical development has been dramatic.

Of the two treatment strategies, checkpoint therapy against **PD-1 has proven more effective,** and positive results are being observed in several types of cancer, including lung cancer, renal cancer, lymphoma, and melanoma. Checkpoint therapy has fundamentally changed the outcome for certain groups of patients with advanced cancer...

Checkpoint therapy has now revolutionized cancer treatment and has fundamentally changed the way we view how cancer can be managed."

CHAPTER FOUR

Discoveries of Nobel Laureate
U.S. Scientist James P. Allison, PhD

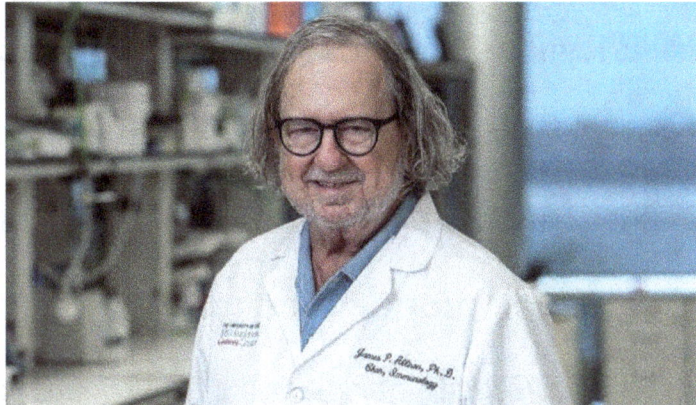

The idea of fighting against cancer by "reactivating" cancer-inactivated natural immunity in patients was **profound.** The survival rate of patients with advanced-stage and metastatic cancers, which were previously deemed to be "death sentences," has been improved dramatically with current clinical practices of checkpoint-inhibiting immunotherapy.

Ipilimumab (Yervoy), an anti-CTLA-4 mAb (monoclonal antibody), was approved as the first Immune Checkpoint Inhibitor by the Food and Drug Administration (FDA) in 2011. Since then, a total of seven types of ICIs targeting CTLA-4 and PD-1/PD-L1, have been approved for cancer immunotherapy in the last decade.

The Immunotherapy Miracle!

In the 1990s, Allison's lab discovered that, **when inhibited**, a molecule on the surface of T-cells called CTLA-4 can cause the body to unleash T cells previously hidden cancer cells, and find, destroy and remember them.

CTLA-4 is a protein-coding gene. It is an inhibitory receptor expressed primarily by T-cells. It regulates the immune system by binding to B7 on the antigen-presenting cancer tumor cell. This turns off the immune system's T-Cell activity, acting as a **brake** that prevents T-cells from attacking cancer cells. Allison's lab developed a "**monoclonal antibody**" to block the CTLA-4/ B-7 signal, which freed T Cells to attack and destroy cancer cells.

Go to this Link: https://www.youtube.com/watch?v=5AXApBbj1ps

Allison assisted in the creation of monoclonal antibodies capable of locking onto CTLA-4s, "switch off this negative immune system signal" to release the brakes on the immune system, to trigger a reactivation of immune cells to annihilate the cancer cells.

Dr. Allison directed Dana Leach, who worked at his lab, to test how blocking CTLA-4 affected the immune response in cancerous tumors.

Leach injected the monoclonal antibody into mice with bowel cancer. The results were profound! Dr Allison later reflected, "When Dana Leach showed me the initial data, I was pleasantly shocked! In **ALL of the tests, the tumors had regressed completely**!"

When tested in mice, he was able to eliminate cancer tumors, and when duplicated in humans, it led to the development of *ipilimumab* (Yervoy), the first CTLA-4 inhibitor drug approved for melanoma by the FDA in 2011.

This led to the development and FDA Approval for the first checkpoint inhibitor, *ipilimumab (Yervoy by Bristol Myers Squibb),* for advanced melanoma and which was later extended for other cancers.

A second negative immune checkpoint inhibitor, PD-1, on the T-Cell was discovered in 2000, named pembrolizumab (Keytruda) and nivolumab (Opdivo), which block the negative checkpoint inhibitor, PD-1, which is on the T Cell. Their discovery, as well as development of the anti-PD-1 monoclonal antibodies (mAbs) has remarkably advanced cancer immunotherapy in treating many cancers, such as metastatic melanoma, non-small-cell lung cancer (NSCLC), head and neck cancer, bladder, kidney, breast, head and neck cancer, Hodgkin lymphoma, and many others.

A third type of immune checkpoint inhibitor blocks PD-L1 on the cancer cell, which is a molecule that triggers the negative immune checkpoint PD-1. These include atezolizumab (Tecentriq), avelumab (Bavencio), and durvalumab (Imfinzi).

Humanizing my Immunotherapy Research

The following inspiring Interview with Jim Allison, PhD, Nobel Prize Recipient for his discoveries in the field of Immunology, was published on the MD Anderson Website. It shows the human value of his work.

"I don't know the exact number of people who've benefitted from ipilimumab, but I do know there are a lot alive today who wouldn't be otherwise.

The first time I met a patient who'd taken ipilimumab was in 2006. I'd been involved in clinical trials for several years. One day, I was in my office, and an oncologist I worked with very closely called and said, 'Hey. Can you come down to the outpatient clinic for a minute? I said, OK. There, he introduced me to a 23-year-old patient who'd been diagnosed with stage IV melanoma the year before. She'd had 31 metastases in her liver and another in her brain and had been told she only had about six months left to live. Then she got a single round of treatment with the drug I developed, and her tumors =completely melted away.

The day I met this woman was her first follow-up visit, and her oncologist had told her there were **no signs of cancer left in her body.** He asked her if she wanted to meet the man who'd made that possible. She did, and we ended up becoming good friends. She's 15 years out from being treated now, and married with two kids — living a rich, vibrant life."

CHAPTER FIVE

Tasuku Honjo and the Discovery of Programmed Cell Death Protein PD-1

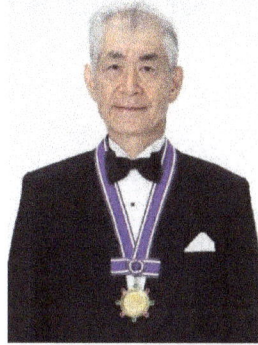

American Research Scientist, James Allison, and Japanese Research Scientist, Tasuku Honjo, showed different strategies for releasing the brakes on the immune system, which could be used to attack cancer cells. "The seminal discovery by the two Laureates constitutes a landmark in our fight against cancer," the Nobel Committee said in a statement.

Following is an Interview with Tasuku Honjo, published in Asian Scientist, June 13, 2016:

"What was your role in the discovery of PD-1?"

"We discovered PD-1 in 1992 when we were looking for something else. So in a way, we accidentally 'bumped into' this molecule.

"We thought that PD-1 protein, which is expressed on activated T cells, was quite interesting, so we went on to study its function.

We deleted the corresponding genes in mice to make knock-out animal models and tried to see what happened. As it turns out, those mice began to exhibit various immune diseases, which suggested that PD-1 was suppressing their immune response. We theorized that by suppressing PD-1, you could boost immune response and hopefully treat cancers that way. That was the starting point: we showed in a study published in 2002 that a *PD-1 blockade can indeed cure cancer in animal models.*

From there, it took another 12 years for us to reach the clinic. In 2014, our anti-PD-1 antibody therapy was approved by the FDA as a drug to treat late-stage melanoma. From discovery to clinical application, it took us 22 years; a long time!"

The Nobel Prize Committee noted that.

"Allison's and Honjo's labs weren't the only ones pursuing checkpoint blockade as an anti-cancer tumor strategy.

However, in 1994, Allison's lab was the only one to demonstrate that mice treated with monoclonal antibodies against CTLA-4 showed a spectacular response, with their tumors disappearing!"

CHAPTER SIX

It Takes a Village to Cure Cancer

CRI Names Winners of Top Scientific Prize

September 3, 2014 - Immune to Cancer: The Cancer Research Institute

Matthew Tontonoz

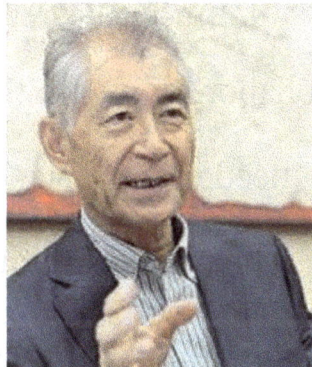

Back in the early 1990s, Tasuku Honjo and his colleagues at Kyoto University were looking to identify genes involved in programmed cell death, a natural process that is part of normal cellular housekeeping.

Through a kind of genetic process of elimination, they identified a gene in cell culture lines that was required for normal programmed cell death. They named this gene, fittingly, programmed cell death-1 (PD-1).

The exact function of PD-1 remained elusive for several years. Clues to its biological function came in 1999 from genetic knock-out experiments in mice, where Sharpe, Honjo, and colleagues disrupted the PD-1 gene and waited to see what would happen.

The Immunotherapy Miracle!

Interestingly, about half of these mice developed a lupus-like syndrome, suggesting that PD-1 was somehow involved in negatively regulating immune function. Lupus is an autoimmune disorder caused by an over-reactive immune system that attacks normal cells.

Further clues to its function came from discovering the natural ligands for the PD-1 receptor, called PD-L1 —work that was accomplished by Arlene Sharpe and Gordon Freeman, in collaboration with the Honjo lab, in 2000 and 2001. By identifying the signals needed to engage the PD-1 pathway, this work provided crucial tools with which to study the pathway and prove its role in negatively regulating T cell function. "Gordon and Arlene closed the loop," said Jim Allison, who chaired the team of CRI scientists and former Coley Award winners who chose this year's recipients.

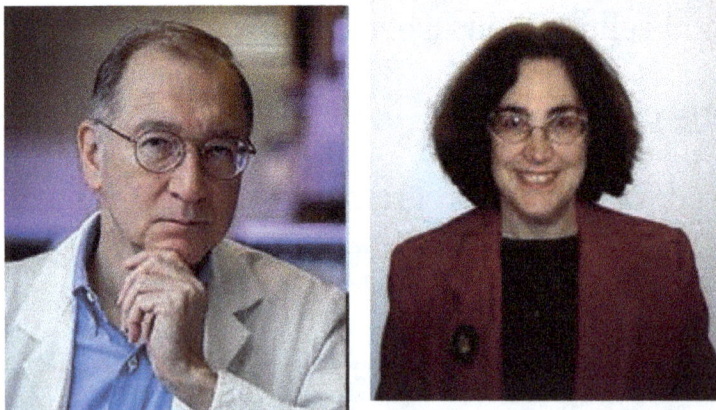

In addition to confirming the immunosuppressive role of the PD-1 pathway, Sharpe and Freeman further noted that their newly identified ligands were found on some cancer cell lines.

This suggested that the PD-1 pathway might play a role in cancer cell tumor evasion of the immune system. 'It is worth noting that PD-L1 and PD-L2 mRNA expression are up-regulated in a variety of tumor cell lines,' they noted in a 2001 *Nature Immunology* article. "These findings give impetus to the investigation of whether PD-L expression on tumors attenuates anti-tumor responses."

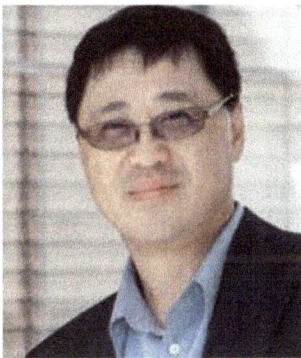

Around the same time that Sharpe and Freeman were identifying the ligands for PD-1, Lieping Chen, then of the Mayo Clinic and now of Yale University, was discovering PD-L1, independently, which he called B7-H1. He went on to make a strong link between B7-H1/PD-L1 and cancer.

In 2002, Chen showed that multiple tumor types express B7-H1/PD-L1, and that PD-L1 on tumors can cause apoptosis (programmed cell death) of tumor-specific T cells.

He further showed that antibodies directed against PD-L1 could lead to tumor rejection.

"These findings have implications for the design of T cell–based cancer immunotherapy," Chen and his colleagues wrote, with significant understatement, in a 2002 Nature Medicine article.

CHAPTER SEVEN

How Checkpoint Inhibitors Reignite The Immune System Against Cancer

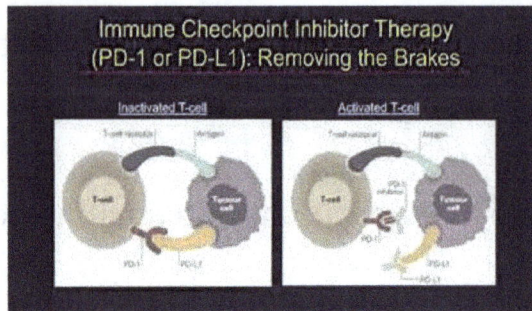

When the **PD-1 negative checkpoint protein** on the **Immune System T-Cell Receptor, connects** to its partner ligand, the **PD-L1 checkpoint protein on the Antigen Presenting Cancer-Tumor Cell**, the **brakes** are put on the immune system, which is **turned off** against the Cancer Cells. This allows the cancer cells to evade or mask themselves from the immune system and proliferate and spread uncontrolled.

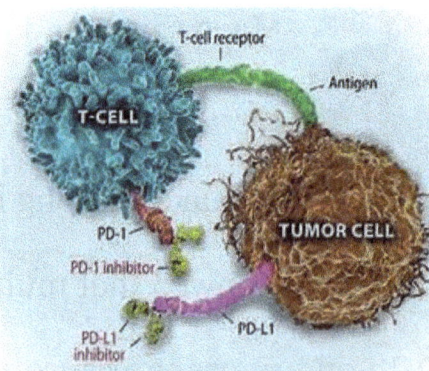

When a monoclonal antibody (mAb) targets, blocks, and prevents binding to a specific checkpoint protein (called a checkpoint blockade), it breaks the connection and, in essence, the accelerator on the immune system is activated. The immune cells are *unleashed!* The Natural Killer Cells, Cytotoxic T-cells, Helper T-cells, Memory T-cells, and other parts of the immune system find, mark, destroy, and remember the cancer cells for future destruction!

The ligand partner protein for CTLA-4, the first discovered negative checkpoint protein on the Immune T-Cell, is checkpoint proteins, B-7-1, 2 on the Cancer-Tumor Cell. It works the same way as the PD-1/PD-L1 checkpoints.

Checkpoint Inhibitor Monoclonal Antibodies

A natural antibody is a Y-shaped protein component produced by the immune system to fight off harmful substances called **antigens**.

One of the best ways of controlling the immune system, with the highest precision, is with ANTIBODIES, which are B-cells produced in the bone marrow. They are on patrol, circulating through the blood, with the mission of recognizing and neutralizing substances that are foreign to the body. The job of the antibody is to lock onto antigens and then destroy or incapacitate them, or to directly flag them for destruction by an immune cell.

Monoclonal Antibodies (mAbs)

One of the most significant discoveries of our time was the invention of lab-made Monoclonal Antibodies, as a partnership of science with nature.

In 1975, Georges Kohler, a German biologist, and Cesar Milstein, an Argentinian biochemist, who later became a British Citizen, published a landmark paper describing a technique for generating a large amount of lab-made monoclonal antibodies, with a pre-defined specificity. For this watershed discovery, they shared a Nobel Prize in Physiology or Medicine in 1984 with Niels Kaj Jerne, who was born in London. Monoclonal Antibodies (mAbs) mimic the functions of natural antibodies within the immune system.

The Immunotherapy Miracle!

Monoclonal antibodies, abbreviated as "mAbs," were developed to *target* a very specific part of a cell, and are an integral part of Checkpoint Inhibitor Immunotherapy.

They are produced from a cell lineage made by cloning a unique white blood cell. All lab-made antibodies derived this way trace back to a unique parent cell. Because it is "mono" clonal, it can only bind to *one* target on the same antigen (epitope).

Different monoclonal antibodies used in immunotherapy, checkpoint inhibitors, such as pembrolizumab (Keytruda) and others, function by blocking the PD-1 receptor on the immune T-Cell or PD-L1 on the antigen-presenting cancer cells. This mechanism, referred to as a "checkpoint blockade," blocks the cellular mechanism that turns back **on** the immune system, and it is a "**checkmate**" for the cancer cells!

While the two linked checkpoints put the brakes on the immune system and hide the cancer cells. The monoclonal "checkpoint inhibitor" acts as a "brake release" and accelerator that reactivates the anti-cancer tumor immune response. This allows the immune system's T-cells and other parts of the immune system to attack and destroy cancer cells! The immune system can find, eliminate, mark, and remember the cancer cells for future destruction.

CHAPTER EIGHT

Immunotherapy Checkpoint Inhibiting Drugs

In recent years, there has been a wave of new miracle cancer-killing drugs available, all ending with the suffix "—mab". Researching this uncovered suffix stands for the source, which is "monoclonal antibody."

The 1 or 2 letters before the source (mab) tell you where in the body the monoclonal antibody has been shown to work. Here's a quick list of the most common targets:

- -c(i)-: circulatory system

- -k(i)-: interleukin

- -l(i)-: immune system

- -t(u)-: tumor

- -u-: human (all human)

- -o-: mouse (all mouse)

- -xi-: chimeric (part human, part nonhuman)

- -zu-: humanized (mostly human)

- -li-: shown to work in the immune system

The Immunotherapy Miracle!

As of August 2025, approximately eleven different types of monoclonal antibody-based checkpoint inhibitors have been produced and FDA-approved since 2011.

The following is a nonexhaustive list of some FDA approvals for immune checkpoint-inhibiting monoclonal antibodies:

Ipilimumab (Yervoy) (blocks CTLA-4)	March 2011
Optivo (Nivolumab)	September 2014
Keytruda (Pembrolizumab)*	December 2014
Libtayo (cemiplimab)	September 2018
Dostarlimab (Jemperli)	April 2021

Among current immunotherapy checkpoint inhibitor options, pembrolizumab (Keytruda) and nivolumab (Opdivo) are widely considered to have the highest success rate in many cancer types, showing significant improvements in overall survival rates compared to standard chemotherapy treatments, with significantly fewer side effects. Opdivo can be combined with Yervoy.

The drug dostarlimab (Jemperli) showed amazing results in Clinical Trials that were instrumental in FDA Approval in 2021. To see News on the 100% Cure of Rectal Cancer Clinical Trial, go to the LINK below:

https://youtu.be/a0rbO3pnqDI

CHAPTER NINE

WARRIORS WITHIN! THE IMMUNE SYSTEM
Finding, Destroying, and Remembering Cancer Cells

Immunotherapy checkpoint inhibitors work by harnessing the body's immune system! Following is a simplified explanation of how immunotherapy activates the Warriors Within to find, flag, destroy, and remember cancer.

White blood cells include lymphocytes, which are T-cells that include CD4 Helper Cells, CD8 Cytotoxic T-cells, Treg Regulatory Cells, Memory Cells, and Killer T-cells, as well as B-cells, which create antibodies. A Lymphocyte can cause an immune response when it identifies "antigens," which are foreign substances in the body.

Other White Blood Cells are natural killer cells, neutrophils, eosinophils, basophils, and monocytes, which are neither T-cells nor B-cells. B-cells are created in the bone marrow and produce natural antibodies. Precursors of T-cells originate in the bone marrow and migrate to the Thymus to mature. T Cells are specifically programmed to recognize and destroy cells with abnormal antigens. This includes cancer cells. Cancer cells have antigens as surface markers that notify the immune system if something in your body is harmful, triggering an immune response.

The Immunotherapy Miracle!

Dendritic Cells recognize the cancer cells as foreign and capture, flag, and present them for the immune system to recognize and destroy.

They function with the assistance of the Helper T-cells (CD-4), which don't directly kill abnormal cells, but instead, release signaling molecules called cytokines to activate other immune cells to destroy them.

In cancer destruction, the major killers of the cancerous tumor cells are cytotoxic T cells (CD8), which are a part of the **adaptive** immune response, and NK (Natural Killer) Cells are a part of the **innate** immune response. Natural Killer Cells can rapidly respond to threats without prior activation to **directly attack and destroy cancer cells**.

Conversely, Cytotoxic T-cells (CD8) must be activated by antigen-presenting cells (the cancer tumor cell). **They can release granules to kill multiple cancerous cells in succession and then move to a new target to kill again, which is often referred to as serial killing.**

Granulocytes, a type of white blood cell, include neutrophils, eosinophils, and basophils, which surround and destroy the abnormal cancer cells through the release of cytotoxic granules containing enzymes and other chemicals. Monocytes can turn into macrophages to destroy and engulf cancer cells. Immune Checkpoint Inhibitors are miraculous because the divine intelligence of the awe-inspiring immune system is miraculous!

CHAPTER TEN

New Immunotherapy Shots!

Source: Express, UK, May 1, 2025. Go to the following website:

https://www.express.co.uk/life-style/health/2049062/new-five-minute-super-jab-nhs-will

New NHS 'Super-Jab' will Treat 15 Cancers and Transform Lives

by Fiona Callingham & Hayley Parker

The NHS (National Health Service, England) is set to roll out a new five-minute 'super-jab' that can treat 15 types of cancer and will 'transform lives'. Thousands of patients in England are set to benefit after the NHS became the first in Europe to offer the injection.

The jab is an injectable form of immunotherapy, nivolumab. This means patients can receive their fortnightly (every two weeks) or monthly treatment in five minutes instead of up to an hour via an IV drip. Officials say it can be used to treat 15 cancer types, including skin, bladder, and esophagus cancer. An estimated 1,200 patients in England per month could benefit. The UK's medicines regulator, the Medicines and Healthcare Products Regulatory Agency (MHRA), approved use of the injection yesterday (April 30, 2025).

The Immunotherapy Miracle!

In clinical trials, the NHS reported that patients were highly satisfied with the under-the-skin injection. They preferred it to the IV form of the drug, which takes 30 to 60 minutes every two to three weeks or four to six weeks, depending on the dosage and cancer type.

Around two in five patients who currently receive IV nivolumab, one of the most widely used cancer treatments, should be eligible for the new jab.

NHS cancer services are now preparing to treat the first patients with the new treatment next month, when supplies of the product are received in the UK.

Professor Peter Johnson, NHS England national clinical director for cancer, said: "Immunotherapy has already been a huge step forward for many NHS patients with cancer, and being able to offer it as an injection in minutes means we can make the process far more convenient."

This treatment is used for 15 different types of cancer, so it will free up thousands of valuable clinicians' time every year, allowing teams to treat even more patients and help increase hospital capacity. Clinical pharmacist and national specialty adviser for cancer drugs, James Richardson, added: 'I am delighted that NHS patients across England will soon be able to benefit from this quick and effective treatment, which can be used to treat a range of cancer types.'

This is a significant advancement in cancer treatment, with the potential to improve the lives of thousands of patients each month".

The faster treatment comes at no extra cost to the NHS due to an agreement between NHS England and the manufacturer Bristol Myers Squibb."

Keytruda's Pembrolizumab Injection is in Clinical Trials And Pending FDA Approval in the U.S.

An injectable version of KEYTRUDA is in the last stage of clinical trials. Merck is seeking FDA approval for a subcutaneous under-the-skin formulation of KEYTRUDA in addition to the currently approved IV form. The goal is to provide a more convenient and potentially accessible treatment option for patients. The FDA has accepted Merck's regulatory filing for the subcutaneous version of KEYTRUDA. A final decision is expected by September 23rd, 2025.

Merck is seeking approval for the subcutaneous (injectable shot) version across all solid tumors for which the drug's intravenous version is already approved. In Stage 3 Trials, it is as effective as the intravenous version. Pending the final approval of the FDA, an injectable shot of pembrolizumab (Keytruda) is expected to be available in the United States on October 1, 2025, to some patients.

CHAPTER ELEVEN

The Back Story of Checkpoint Inhibitor Discovery

One of my favorite College courses was entitled "The Advancement of Scientific Thought". It showed how one Scientific discovery was necessary to provide the foundational information for the next. On this principle, it took a Village of inspired Research Scientists compounding on previous discoveries to find the curative answer to cancer.

It was not until April 14, 2003, that the *'International Human Genome Sequencing Consortium'* announced the completion of the Human Genome Project, which mapped and sequenced the genes. The *genome* is the entire set of DNA instructions found in a cell. This created research tools to allow scientists to identify genes involved in disease and the regulation of the immune system, through new tools such as gene cloning and gene knockoffs.

Also, the monumental discovery of T-cells and B-cells was not made until the mid-1960s and early 1970s

Additionally, the subtypes of white blood cells, such as Cytotoxic T Cells, Memory T-cells, Helper T-cells, and Suppressor T-cells, which were the organizing principle of the adaptive immune system, were not discovered until the mid-1970s.

The following is from an October 30, 2023, Interview with Gordon Freeman, PhD, regarding the backstory leading up to the profound Discovery of the "Checkpoint Blockade" that unleashes the Immune System to find, flag, destroy, and remember cancer cells!

Upon finishing his Doctorate in 1979 at the renowned Dana Farber Cancer Institute in Boston, Gordon Freeman, PhD, decided that the most exciting area of science, ready to open up, was *immunology*.

Freeman decided to pursue his first post-doctorate with Harvey Cantor, MD, as his Mentor. Freeman called him an "Immunology Star at Dana Farber." While Cantor did not discover T-cells, Cantor was recognized for his significant contributions to the development and understanding of the different immunological functions of the subsets of T-cells. These included the characterization of regulatory T Cells (Tregs), which play a critical role in maintaining immune tolerance and preventing autoimmune diseases, as well as additional T-Cell subtype classifications such as Cytotoxic T Cells, Memory T-cells, and Helper T-cells.

Significantly, during Freeman's post-doc with Harvey Cantor, in his path toward the implementation of Immune Checkpoint Inhibitors, he learned how to apply molecular biology and gene cloning to T cells.

Freeman then did a second post-doc with Lee Nadler, a pioneer in identifying the markers in B cells. He had markers that he called B-1, B-2, B-3, and Nadler, and Freeman was working on one called B-7. Freeman was the molecular biologist who cloned the B7 molecule. Crucially, Nadler and Freeman found that B-7 was the major signal for co-stimulating T cells and that it was necessary for T cells to grow and expand.

Next, Freeman became an Assistant Professor at the Dana Farber Institute and started a lab of his own during the days when the human genome was being sequenced, and 20,000 new genes became available to study.

Freeman looked for the molecular cousins of the B7 molecule, believing that they would be significantly important to regulating the immune system.

Because of his postdoc experience with mentors who were among the top immunologists in the world, Freeman was able to bring molecular biology and Gene Cloning to the lab, which led them to the discovery of molecules that we now know as PD-1 and PD-L1.

Freeman worked with Clive Wood and Tasuku Honjo and, to their amazement, showed that PD-L1 was a ligand for the PD-1 molecule, and this PD-L1/PD-1 pathway turned off the T-cells and immune response.

In Gordon Freeman's own words,

"The surprising thing was that we discovered PD-L1 in cancer cells, so we went and looked at where it was expressed and, to our surprise, it was expressed on the surface of solid tumor cancer cells.

We thought we'd find it on immune cells like dendritic cells and macrophages, but this was a molecule that cancer cells were using, and they were sort of stealing its function and using it to turn off the Immune System T-Cell early in response.

I came to the Dana Farber Institute because I thought it was a world leader in immunology, and I thought that the power of the immune system could be used to fight cancer. I believed that was a really good idea because your immune system can learn and change, and adapt. I thought if you could bring that power against cancer, it could change how we treat cancer.

Around the year 2000, three incredible strands of research started at the Dana Farber. The discovery of the PD-L1/PD-1 pathway led to successful immunotherapy. If the patients who responded were alive after two years, they continued to be alive for many more years, and when you looked 10 years forward. The great majority of the patients who were OK at two years were still alive at 10 years, so immunotherapy was different. **It was leading to durable long-term effects, which optimists would call a cure**."

I think we first realized how impressive the PD-L1 /PD-1 therapy was at the 2012 meeting of the ASCO Society, the American Society of Clinical Oncology.

(NOTE: ASCO's Mission is, "Conquering cancer through research, education, and promotion of the highest quality of patient care."

ASCO's Goal is: "A world where cancer is prevented and cured and every survivor is healthy.")

They have over 20,000 members and hold a large conference each year, where cancer doctors come together to hear about the latest developments. There was a session in a large, packed room, and three speakers essentially stated that the PD-L1/PD-1 therapy would be effective in Melanoma. Lung and kidney cancer, this was just the dawn of a revolution. The excitement in that hall was incredible!

My mother was a heavy smoker and died of lung cancer. She passed in a matter of months. One of the thrills of my scientific career is that this works in lung cancer. I was lucky to have one of the nurses call me and say that there was a patient who wanted to meet me as one of the pioneers in the field of checkpoint inhibitors. I got together with her patient, Barry Nelson.
Barry had lung cancer and was told he should head for hospice.
After Immunotherapy, Barry is still alive 10 years later and is doing well.

It's been an incredible thrill to get to know a patient for whom this has worked. I only wish it had come 10 years earlier.

This is a "family business." I've worked with my wife, Arlene Sharpe, on cancer immunotherapy for almost 35 years. It used to be that the family business was that I would discover the molecule and then her lab over at

Harvard Medical School would knock it out, helping to determine its function in the body."

INTERVIEW with Arlene Sharpe, PhD

"I never imagined when this (PD1/ PD-L1) pathway was discovered that it would have a biology that was so broad and important in cancer. It turns out that this pathway has been chosen, over and over again, by cancers as well as microbes that cause chronic infection as a means to inhibit anti-tumor immunity. So, antibodies that block PD1 or that black PD-L1 have been developed, so you're blocking the interaction between the ligand and the receptor to block that inhibitory signal, so when the signal is blocked, those T cells can work better, you're raising the veil of immunosuppression and releasing the brakes. Now you have good anti-tumor immunity. Early studies were done in several tumors in melanoma and lung cancer, and now we know that this pathway is effective in blocking this pathway in over 30 different cancer cell types, so it has broad effects."

CHAPTER TWELVE

Gordon Freeman, PhD, and Arlene Sharpe, PhD
Husband and Wife, Immunotherapy Dynamic Duo!

Gordon Freeman, PhD, Associate Professor of Medicine, Department of Medical Oncology at the Dana-Farber Cancer Institute, and Arlene Sharp, MD, PhD, the distinguished Kolokotrones University Professor at Harvard University and Chair of the Department of Immunology at Harvard Medical School, a married couple joined forces and made groundbreaking discoveries in Immunology Checkpoint Inhibitors, which were foundational in the development of cancer immunotherapy drugs like the PD-1 Inhibitors pembrolizumab (*Keytruda*, Merck & Co) and nivolumab (*Optivo*, Bristol-Myers Squibb).

At the beginning of their research, Research Scientists Freeman and Arlene Sharpe worked together at their respective labs at the Dana Farber Cancer Institute and Harvard Medical School, trying to discover which genes, out of approximately 20,000, control the immune system.

Freeman cloned particular genes that he believed were instrumental in immune function, and Sharpe used a tool called "gene knockout" to see the gene's function.

The "knockout" would eliminate the suspected gene (knock it out) to determine how the body would react without it.

Significantly, Shape, PhD, and her lab made a pivotal discovery that CTLA-4 was an **inhibitory** "negative checkpoint" that acts as a "brake" that keeps the immune system in "check." The cancer cells had commandeered the newly discovered molecular pathway that allowed them to hide from the immune system.

Sharpe made a pivotal discovery, finding that CTLA-4 acted as a "brake" that keeps the immune system in "check" and stops it from functioning, and when that "brake" was taken off, the immune system goes into "attack mode!"

Their discoveries led to the development of drugs known as "checkpoint inhibitors," which mobilize the body's immune system to attack cancerous tumors, which were previously hiding from the immune system. Popular immunotherapy treatments, such as *pembrolizumab (Keytruda),* which allows the immune system to destroy cancerous tumors, and *ipilimumab* (Yervoy), which treats advanced melanoma, have become an alternative to surgery, chemotherapy, and radiation for cancer patients.

Significantly, the discoveries of Arlene Sharpe helped identify the key targets for immunotherapy and their functions.

Additionally, Gordon Freeman, Sharpe, and their labs found a pathway similar to the CTLA-4 pathway between the PD-1 checkpoint on the

T-cells, and the PD-L1 checkpoint on the cancer cell tumor. When this pathway was connected, it allowed the cancer cells to hijack the immune system to keep them from recognizing and eliminating them.

They further found that blocking that connection with a monoclonal antibody checkpoint inhibitor can unleash the immune system to discover, destroy, and remember the cancer cells.

In summary, Freeman, Sharpe, and their labs showed that PD-L1 binds to PD-1 to turn off the immune response to cancer, and that a blockade of the PD-1/PD-L1 signal enhanced the immune response.

They showed that PD-1 is expressed on many cancerous tumors, allowing them to resist immune attack.

A Clinical 1 Trial showed pembrolizumab (Keytruda), a fully humanized anti-PD-1 monoclonal antibody, was found in clinical studies to be safe and effective for the treatment of melanoma.

A Phase II Clinical Trial showed that the curative effect of pembrolizumab for advanced melanoma was obvious when compared with that of ipilimumab (an anti-CTLA-4 antibody).

THE PROFOUND "AHA" MOMENTS

Both CTLA-4 (cytotoxic T-lymphocyte-related protein) and PD-1 (programmed death ligand-1) are the negative regulators of immune responses. A "negative regulator" is a protein on the surface of an immune cell that acts to suppress the immune response by inhibiting T Cell activation.

CTLA-4 or PD-1, expressed on the surface of activated T cells, forces T cells to ignore cancer cells. PD-1 attracted a molecule now known as PD-L1, its ligand. Crucially, it was discovered that cancerous cells often produce PD-L1. "The first ones we found were on ovarian and breast cancer cells," says Freeman.

"Then, we found it on lots of other cancer cells and realized that PD-L1 (programmed death ligand-1) seemed to be the trick, cancers used to turn on the immune brake.

The immune system Checkpoint inhibitors are a type of immunotherapy that utilizes lab-made monoclonal antibodies to block proteins that are responsible for hiding cancer cells from the immune system.

Freeman and Sharpe showed that PD-L1 is highly expressed on many cancerous tumors, which allows them to resist immune attack, and **that a blockade of the signal between PD-L1 to PD-1 reignited cancer-killing immune responses**.

Crucially, they also discovered that cancerous cells often produce PD-L1. "The first ones we found were on ovarian and breast cancer cells," says Freeman. **"Then, we found it on lots of other cancer cells and**

realized that PD-L1 seemed to be the trick cancer used to turn OFF the immune system! That was the 'aha' moment."

What Freeman, Honjo, and their teams had discovered is that PD-L1 on the surface of cancer cells allied with PD-1. This called off the immune attack, allowing cancer to proliferate unchallenged. So, could blocking PD-1 stymie cancer? To test the idea, Honjo tried growing human tumors in mice that were genetically engineered to lack PD-1 on their surface.

To restore the suppressed ability of immune cells to recognize cancer cells, Monoclonal antibodies (mAbs) have been adopted as immune checkpoint inhibitors (ICIs) by blocking the PD-1/PD-L1 interactions of immune checkpoints between cancer and immune cells.

In 2014, Freeman received the _William B. Coley Award_ along with Arlene Sharpe, Tasuku Honjo, and Lieping Chen.

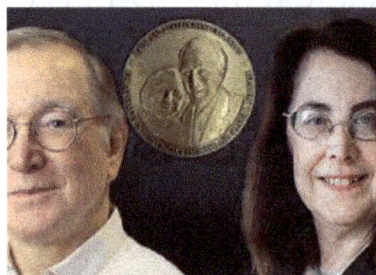

In 2017, Gordon Freeman and Arlene Sharpe also won the prestigious _"Warren Alpert Foundation Prize"_ along with Lieping Chen, James P. Allison, and Tasuku. Honjo, for their collective contributions to the pre-clinical foundation and development of the immune checkpoint blockade and for their breakthrough work identifying costimulatory pathways that control the

activation and inhibition of T cell immune responses, leading to new, effective

immunotherapies for cancer, autoimmune diseases, and transplant rejection."

News > Medscape Medical News > Oncology News'
The 'Family Business' Behind the Flurry of PD-1 Inhibitors
Alexander M. Castellino, PhD
September 10, 2014

"Meet the husband-and-wife team of Gordon Freeman, PhD, Associate

Professor of Medicine, Department of Medical Oncology at the Dana-

Farber Cancer Institute, and Arlene Sharp, MD, PhD, the distinguished

Kolokotrones University Professor at Harvard University Medical

School, and Chair of the Department of Immunology, who were crucial

in assembling pieces of this immunotherapy puzzle.

"I joke that it's the family business," Dr. Freeman told *Medscape*

Medical News about their shared research focus. Discoveries from the

couple's respective labs have been translated into therapies that are

changing the face of cancer treatment.

Doctors Freeman and Sharpe patented the PD-1/PD-L1 pathway

first, but allowed their intellectual property to be non-exclusively

distributed.

For Dr. Freeman, the PD-1 story dates back to the 1980s,

specifically to 1987, when a molecule called *B7 — the seventh antigen on B cells* — was discovered. B7 belongs to a family of ligands that activate T cells.

With the completion of the Human Genome Project, Dr. Freeman and his colleagues investigated the database for other sequences that were similar to B7 sequences and discovered PD-L1.

Any telling of the story of the development of PD inhibitors should include Japan. That's where Tasuku Honjo, MD, PhD, from Kyoto University School of Medicine and its colleagues first identified the PD-1 molecule in the 1990s. Honjo won a Nobel Prize in 2018, along with James Allison, PhD.

In a collaboration, which included Clive R. Wood, PhD, then at the Genetics Institute and Wyeth Research, and Dr. Honjo, Dr. Freeman showed that the PD-1/PD-L1 interaction resulted in negative regulation of lymphocyte activation. **'It turns off the immune response and provides a drug target**,' Dr. Freeman said.

Simultaneously, PD-L1 was independently discovered by Lieping Chen, MD, PhD, then of Mayo Clinic in Rochester, Minnesota, and now at Yale University in New Haven, Connecticut, who also offered insights into its significance.

According to Dr. Freeman, "Work on PD-1 was a watershed moment for pharmaceutical development." He explained that the PD-1 pathway started as a basic lab discovery and has now really taken off. "We've cured cancer 50 ways in mice, and PD-1 is what works well in people," he added.

Drug development on the first PD-1 inhibitor, *nivolumab,* was accomplished by Alan Korman's team at Medarex, a biotech company with research facilities in California that was acquired by Bristol-Myers Squibb in 2009.

The PD-1 inhibitors seem to reverse tumor escape from immune surveillance across several cancers, including melanoma, lung, bladder, and kidney cancers, and Hodgkin lymphoma. These cancers are being targeted with PD-1 inhibitors used alone or in combination with other inhibitors that target specific pathways associated with tumor proliferation.

On September 4, 2014, the US Food and Drug Administration approved Merck's drug *pembrolizumab* for patients with advanced melanoma. Moreover, *nivolumab*, another PD-1 inhibitor from Bristol-Myers Squibb and Ono Pharmaceutical, was first approved in Japan.

In Dr. Arlene Sharpe's lab on the Harvard campus, other pieces of the puzzle were being assembled. 'Early on, PD-L1 was intriguing because we wanted to understand what differentiates it from B7,' she told *Medscape Medical News*.

In a collaboration with Rafi Ahmed, PhD, at the Emory University School of Medicine, Dr. Sharpe and Dr. Freeman, and their colleagues showed that PD-1 belongs to a family of molecules, which includes CTLA4 (the target for ipilimumab).

The excitement mounted when the husband-and-wife duo discovered PD-L1 tumor cells had learned how to hijack the PD-1 receptor on immune T cells. The PD-1/PD-L1 interaction in the tumor microenvironment turns off the immune response so crucial to tumor recognition and elimination. Blocking PD-1 or PD-L1 using monoclonal antibodies developed in Dr. Freeman's lab **had a dramatic effect: The T cells revived and assumed their normal role."**

CHAPTER THIRTEEN

Contributions of Lieping Chen, PhD

One of the Scientific Researchers who made a major contribution to immunotherapy checkpoint inhibitors was Lieping Chen, M.D, PhD, a Chinese-American immunologist and Physician-Scientist and Co-Director of the Cancer Immunology Program at Yale University. Chen began his teaching career at the Johns Hopkins University of Medicine in 2004 and joined the Yale University School of Medicine in 2010.

When Lieping Chen, M.D., PhD, was training to be an oncologist in the 1980s, he stated, "The lack of effective cancer treatments made it a depressing job. That's why I quit clinical practice," he says. But Chen soon shifted to research focusing on the role of the immune system in cancer.

In 1999, Chen's group at the Mayo Clinic in Rochester, Minnesota, discovered a checkpoint in the B7 family that they named B7-H1.

Chen's laboratory first cloned B7-H-1 (PD-L1), discovered its immune suppressive functions, and demonstrated the role of the PD-1/B-7-H-1 pathway in the evasion of tumor immunity. At this time, Chen was unaware that B7-H1 was PD-L1, which was later determined to be the ligand of PD-1.

Chen discovered that it had the power to suppress the activity of T-cells, but **he did not know the T-cell molecule responsible for this effect.**

The Immunotherapy Miracle!

In 2000 researchers from Harvard's Medical School (Arelene Sharpe), The Dana-Farber Cancer Institute (Gordon Freeman), and the University of Kyoto (Tasuku Honjo) found that B7-H1, which had been renamed PD-L1 **binds to another protein called PD-1,** which was a checkpoint receptor on the surface of T-cells which, when connected with its ligand, renamed PD-L1, suppresses the activity of the T-cells against cancer.

Tasuku Honjo, the Gordon Freeman laboratory, Arlene Sharpe, plus others, identified the ligand for PD-1, without realizing it to be the same protein as Chen's B7-H1, and so named it programmed death-ligand 1 (PD-L1).

Bringing this full circle, Chen, as well as Honjo, Freeman, Sharpe, and their labs, showed that blocking the interaction between PD-1 and PD-L1 by monoclonal antibodies ignited the immune system's ability to eliminate cancer tumors.

Dr. Chen also initiated and helped organize the first human clinical trials of anti-PD-1/PD-L1 antibodies for treating human cancer in 2006 at Johns Hopkins Medical Institute.

CHAPTER FOURTEEN
CONCLUSION

By Lynne Meredith

This book was written to increase "IMMUNOTHERAPY CHECKPOINT INHIBITOR AWARENESS" by utilizing education to reach the critical mass of people worldwide to make this option common knowledge through education.

The IMMUNOLOGY MIRACLE is based upon knowledge that the author gained from saving her own life from metastatic Stage IV cancer, to help others escape the terror, devastation, and heartbreak of cancer.

Immunotherapy checkpoint inhibitors saved her from stage IV cancer and the death sentence given by the oncologists, after a rare and very aggressive cancer (leiomyosarcoma) had spread throughout her bones, liver, and skull. She went from intense pain, unable to roll over in bed, unable to walk, confined to a wheelchair, losing her hearing in her right ear, and rapidly losing 20 pounds...to being cancer-free, pain-free, walking again, able to hear again, and back to a healthy weight!

Sadly, even though Immunotherapy Checkpoint Inhibitors are Nobel Prize-winning, FDA-approved, and recognized as the Fourth Standard of Cancer Care—many still recommend systemic chemotherapy that poisons the body and damages the immune system, with hellacious side effects.

Chemo does not eliminate the Cancer Stem Cells (Cancer Seeds), and in many cases, the tumor metastasizes, making chemo ineffective. Immunotherapy Checkpoint Inhibitors are targeted treatments that specifically attack cancer cells, maintaining a memory of the cancer to eliminate it if it returns.

This book shares the history of immunotherapy checkpoint inhibitors.

It also celebrates the inspired, brilliant scientists who made these discoveries and provides inspiration to others by sharing the stories of the people who received a second chance at life because of them.

The following chapters also introduce science- and research-based discoveries aimed at improving the effectiveness of Immunotherapy Checkpoint Inhibitors with the goal of achieving a 100% cancer cure rate.

Knowledge is power, and knowledge that saves lives is a Superpower. Please share this book, and **GO TELL THE OTHERS!**

"Cancer is indeed one of the darkest battles we face as human beings, and this book shines a luminous light of hope, courage, healing, and empowerment into that shadow. It demonstrates a dedication to giving a voice and power to those fighting for their lives and is nothing short of heroic. Readers will carry this message with them to others long after the final page is turned."

- Marianne Williamson

PART TWO

ENHANCING THE EFFICACY OF IMMUNOTHERAPY CHECKPOINT INHIBITORS

CHAPTER FIFTEEN

Enhancing the Success of Checkpoint Inhibiting Immunotherapy Starts in the *Gut Microbiome*

Harvard Office of Technology Development
April 6th, 2017

70% of Your Immune Function is in Your Gut!

"The gut microbiome is the collection of trillions of microbes that live in the human digestive tract, in the stomach, and small and large intestines, which play a vital role in digestion, immunity, and overall health. It is a complex ecosystem of microbes that colonize the gut.

Combining cutting-edge insights from gut microbiology, immunology, and oncology, Arlene Sharpe, MD, PhD, and Dennis Kasper, MD, are deploying a new 'immune-oncology-microbiome' (IOME) platform to identify new strategies and molecular candidates to improve the outcomes of cancer immunotherapy.

"It has become clear through clinical experience with checkpoint inhibitors that the composition of the microbiome has a strong effect on patients' response to the (checkpoint inhibiting) drugs," said Michal Preminger, Executive Director of Harvard OTD's HMS branch.

The Miracle of the Probiotic, Akkermansia Muciniphilia

Research has shown that probiotic **Akkermansia** levels, which improve anti-tumor effects, is a key player in enhancing the effectiveness of immunotherapy.

Foods that stimulate it include cranberries, concord grapes, and pomegranate juice.

These two pioneering Harvard scientists are now coming together to tackle the riddle of what, in the microbiome, is causing this differential response. "This is a relatively new area of investigation, but the impact of the microbiome on the immune system is dramatic," said Sharpe. "We're just beginning to appreciate the extent to which it controls immune responses… We're excited to have this opportunity to make a substantial contribution to the field and, we hope, to patient care."

"The importance of supporting your microbiome is vital for maximizing immune function because **70% of your immune cells are in your gut**," says David Herber, MD, PhD, and Professor Emeritus of Medicine at UCLA Health. **Nutrition is a key modulator of immune function**."

The immune cells are in a region that is known as the 'Gut Associated Lymphoid Tissue' (GALT). This is a prominent part of Mucosal-Associated Lymphoid Tissue (MALT). Accordingly, more than two-thirds of your body's immune cells reside in the gut. Also, about 80% of plasma cells (mainly immunoglobulin IgA) reside in the GALT. The immune cells in the intestinal wall are organized into specific structures called **Peyer's patches** that are in the **lamina propria** and submucosa of the GI tract. They contain numerous immune cells such as macrophages, DCs, T Cells, and immunoglobulins.

Activation of Natural Killer Cells by Probiotics

Nabil Aziz [1], Benjamin Bonavida [1,*]

Aziz N, Bonavida B. Activation of Natural Killer Cells by Probiotics. For Immunopathol Dis Therap. 2016;7(1-2):41-55. doi: 10.1615/ForumImmunDisTher.2016017095. PMID: 28616355; PMCID: PMC5467532

"Critical to the functions (of the gut microbiome) is to synthesize amino acids and vitamins and extract energy from polysaccharides that are not absorbable. Furthermore, these microorganisms **support the activity of the immune system**. The majority of bacteria present in this gut environment consists of the Gram-positive species **lactobacilli and bifidobacteria.**

Probiotics implement the activation of NK cells and their secretion of immune factors (e.g., interferon-γ, tumor necrosis factor-α, interleukin-2, etc.) and enhance immunotherapy.

Probiotics also interact with the **lamina propria**, a thin layer of tissue in the middle of the mucosa gut wall that influences the immune system. They can also interact with and stimulate various immune cells, including dendritic cells, macrophages, and B and T lymphocytes.

Diet plays a crucial role in shaping the gut microbiome and, therefore, the immune system, as well as the enhancement of immunotherapy against cancer cells. Conversely, a diet high in processed, manmade foods, processed sugar, and unhealthy fats and oils can negatively affect the immune system.

PROBIOTICS
Live Microbes Feed the Gut Biome

Good choices of fermented foods that feed the microbiome are yogurt, kefir (which has five times as many microbes as yogurt), cheeses, sauerkraut, kimchi (a Korean dish made from garlic, cabbage, and chili), kombucha, and soybean-based products such as soy sauce, tempeh, and natto. You can also take probiotic Supplements such as *Lactobacillus* and *Bifidobacterium*.

MEET YOUR PROBIOTICS

LACTOBACILLUS ACIDOPHILUS
This strain is beneficial to your small intestine, where it helps digest food, produce vitamins, and facilitate easy digestion. Lactobacillus acidophilus has been shown to produce lactase (break down milk) and help prevent diarrhea in adults, making it a great addition to this supplement.

BIFIDOBACTERIUM LACTIS
Great for breaking down lactic acid and boosting the general health of your immune system, Bifidobacterium lactis has been shown to support healthy cholesterol levels, and helps in the overall digestion of sugars, fibers, and other macronutrients.

LACTOBACILLUS BREVIS
A natural anti-inflammatory, the benefits of Lactobacillus Brevis are vast. Specifically, this powerful probiotic benefits the human digestive system, supporting digestive health in a number of ways. Some research indicates its ability to combat ulcers. It can also be used to treat urinary tract infections, as well as vaginitis.

LACTOBACILLUS CASEI
This little probiotic pacts a powerful punch against harmful bacteria. It has been show nto lower pH levels in the digestive system and impedes the growth of harmful bacteria, while improving and promoting digestion.

LACTO-BACILLUS PLANTARUM
Found naturally in pickles, kimchi, and other fermented vegetables, Lacto-bacillus plantarum is one of nature's most versatile probiotics, and has been used to treat IBS, and ease the symptoms of Crohn's disease. It's also one of the most antibiotic resistant probiotics, which is key if you're recovering from the use of antibiotics. Some research has shown it may be highly-effective in preventing soy related allergies.

LACTOBACILLUS RHAMNOSUS
A powerful probiotic, Lactobacillus rhamnosus shown in some studies to have the ability to stop allergic reactions to peanuts in 80% of children tested. It has also shown the ability to prevent rotavirus diarrhea in children, along with other various types of diarrhea in both adults and children. This powerful probiotic is perfect for those looking for help with IBS. According to the British Journal of Nutrition in 2013 it may even help increase weight-loss in woman.

Prebiotics that Feed Probiotics

Prebiotics feed probiotics, which are the beneficial bacteria in the gut that promote a healthy microbiome, by nourishing the gut microbes. Prebiotics contribute to digestive health, nutrient absorption, immune function, and mental well-being, and enhance the efficacy of immunotherapy.

Prebiotics are non-digestible carbohydrates that travel to the colon, where they are fermented by gut bacteria. This fermentation process produces beneficial byproducts like short-chain fatty acids, which provide energy for cells and influence various aspects of health.

Prebiotic Foods

- Bananas
- Berries
- Onions
- Garlic
- Leeks
- Asparagus
- lentils
- Artichokes
- Soybeans
- Fiber-Rich Food
- Whole grains
- Legumes
- Beans
- Cabbage
- Mushrooms
- Broccoli
- Avocados
- Cauliflower
- Brussel Sprouts
- Oats
- Sweet Potatoes
- Brussel Sprouts
- Whole-grain rice
- Corn
- Asparagus
- Celery
- Carrots
- Spinach
- Kale
- Buckwheat
- Soybeans
- Artichokes
- Salad Greens
- Whole grains
- Seaweed
- Beets
- Lentils
- Split Peas
- Whole Grain Foods
- Vegetables
- Chia Seeds
- Jerusalem artichokes
- Dandelion greens
- Barley
- Flaxseed
- Burdock Root
- Wheat Bran

Your Second Brain – Located in the Gut!

There is an often-overlooked network of neurons lining the gut called the Enteric Nervous System (ENS) or "the Second Brain!" It is a complex neural network that controls the absorption and digestion of foods and nutrients, and health. It also contains over 100 million nerve cells and neurons. It plays a crucial role in the immune system.

Surprisingly, your gut also contains neurotransmitters. According to Emeran Mayer, professor of physiology, psychiatry, and biobehavioral sciences at the David Geffen School of Medicine at the University of California, Los Angeles (U.C.L.A.), the enteric nervous system, also called the second brain in the gut, uses more than 30 neurotransmitters, including dopamine and serotonin. 95 percent of the body's serotonin is found in the bowels." It underlies the feeling of 'butterflies in the stomach,' 'gut-feelings,' 'gut-wrenching,' and 'stomach-dropping fear.' It releases enzymes for digestion and impacts mood, mental wellness, stress levels, and overall health and immunity.

CHAPTER SIXTEEN

Enhancing Immunotherapy Through ANTIHISTAMINES

As cancer cells are destroyed, they release their contents, which can include HISTAMINE. Research has shown that antihistamines, which block histamines, can enhance responses to immunotherapy by reducing immunosuppression, enhancing T-Cell activity, and reversing side effects.

When Researchers blocked the histamine receptor, HRH1, either by knocking out the gene or with the use of antihistamines, there was increased T-cell activation that stopped tumor growth.

Immunotherapy checkpoint inhibitors have typically been shown to have either no side effects or generally minor or manageable ones. The most common side effects can include itching, skin rash, muscle aches, joint pain, fatigue, and gastrointestinal issues such as diarrhea or loose stools. These same symptoms can be related to an over-release of histamine or histamine intolerance and can be the result of cancer cells being destroyed, which can indicate that the immunotherapy is working. Studies have shown that these side effects can be reversed or lessened with over-the-counter antihistamines.

H1 antihistamines have also been shown to enhance the effects of immunotherapy positively.

Examples of H-1 Antihistamines:

Fexofenadine (Allegra) (generally considered to cause the least drowsiness).
Citirzine (Zyrtec)
Loratadine (Claritin)
Deslorataine (Clarinex)
Levocetirizine (Xyzel)

Antihistamines Can Reverse Side Effects and Improve the Efficacy of Immunotherapy

Researchers found that cancer patients with low plasma histamine levels had a higher overall response rate to PD-1 checkpoint inhibitors compared with patients who had high histamine levels. However, this can be reversed by H-1 Antihistamines.

Remarkably, in mice experiments histamine-deficient tumor cells exhibited reduced tumor growth and enhanced CD8+ T (cytotoxic killer cell) function. Supporting these findings, blood histamine levels in cancer patients before anti-PD-1 checkpoint inhibitor immunotherapy inversely correlated with their response to treatment.

These results indicate that blood histamine concentrations may serve as a biomarker for response to immunotherapy, and H₁ antihistamine may be used as an adjunct for immune checkpoint blockade therapy.

Cancer Health
<u>SCIENCE NEWS</u>

Antihistamines May Improve Response to Immunotherapy
January 27, 2022 • By <u>Sukanya Charuchandra</u>
<u>https://www.cancerhealth.com/article/antihistamines-may-improve-response-immunotherapy</u>

Studies show that H1 antihistamines, which block histamine from binding to H1 receptors, can improve the efficacy of cancer immunotherapy, particularly immune checkpoint inhibitors, helping to explain differences in treatment response. Dihua Yu, MD, PhD, of the University of Texas MD Anderson Cancer Center, and colleagues found that over-the-counter antihistamines—that block histamine receptor H1 (HRH1)— and patients with less histamine in their blood were three times more likely to respond to checkpoint inhibitors.

"Our preclinical findings suggest that antihistamines have the potential to enhance responses to immunotherapy, especially in those with high levels of histamine in the blood," said Yu. **Preclinical studies have shown that blocking these histamine receptors with over-the-counter antihistamines restores T-cell activation and curbs tumor growth.**

The Immunotherapy Miracle!

Antihistamines, often used to treat allergies, are associated with better response to checkpoint inhibitor immunotherapy and improved overall survival, according to study results published in the publication <u>Cancer Cell</u>. Antihistamines were also associated with significantly improved outcomes in immunotherapy patients," Dihua Yu, MD, PhD, of the University of Texas MD Anderson Cancer Center, said in a press release.

Researchers analyzing data from the Cancer Genome Atlas noted that both histamine and the H1 receptor (HRH1, which binds to histamine in humans) were present at high levels within the cancer tumor microenvironment. The HRH1 receptor was highly expressed on certain types of macrophages that suppress immune response, and histamine was present in cancer cells.

While histamine levels increased in parallel with tumor growth, **this could be countered with antihistamines.**

"Our preclinical findings suggest that antihistamines have the potential to enhance responses to immunotherapy, especially in those *with high levels of histamine in the blood*," said Yu.

In a separate set of experiments, Researchers discovered a link between plasma histamine levels and the response to immunotherapy in people with cancer.

Taken together, these findings suggest that pre-existing allergies or high histamine levels can lead to tamped-down immunotherapy response and that antihistamines can significantly enhance the immunotherapy response.

Antihistamines can also alleviate the side effects in those who are sensitive to the histamine release resulting from the destruction of the cancer cells.

Histamine—a chemical released by certain immune cells—causes allergic reactions and plays a role in immune response.

Excess histamine can activate Mast cells, which are immune cells that are a part of your body's defense system and are found in connective tissues throughout the body, especially in the skin and intestines.

Additionally, histamines can also be found in the synovium (the tissue lining of the inner surface of the joint capsules) and tendon sheaths, which are responsible for producing synovial fluid, which is a thick, sticky, jelly-like substance that lubricates and nourishes joints and cartilage.

In summary, retrospective analyses showed that cancer patients who took antihistamines during immunotherapy treatment had significantly improved progression-free survival from cancer.

The Immunotherapy Miracle!

Source:

The Impact of Antihistamines on Immunotherapy: A Systematic Review

Stephanie Nagy [1], Oksana Denis [1], Atif Hussein [2], Marc M Kesselman [1]

February 21, 2025

Nagy S, Denis O, Hussein A, Kesselman MM. The Impact of Antihistamines on Immunotherapy: A Systematic Review. Cureus. 2025 Feb 21;17(2):e79421. doi: 10.7759/cureus 79421. PMID: 40130115; PMCID: PMC11930787. https://pubmed.ncbi.nlm.nih.gov/40130115/

"Recently, the potential interaction between antihistamines and immunotherapies has gained attention. Six articles were included that analyzed this association. In total, 4,171 patients were analyzed with a mean age of 63. Cancer types vary between lungs (including small-cell and non-small-cell lung cancer), melanoma, hepatobiliary, head and neck, breast, gastrointestinal, renal cell, gynecological, and colon cancers. Among all studies, checkpoint inhibitors were used as a form of immunotherapy.

All articles found a significant improvement in overall survival rates and longer progression-free rates when antihistamines were added to immunotherapy regimens compared to patients who did not utilize antihistamines. Additionally, some studies also analyzed mortality rates, and each found a significant reduction in mortality rates when antihistamines were paired with immunotherapy."

Source:

Cancer Cell

Volume 40, Issue 1, 36 - 52.e9

The Allergy Mediator Histamine Confers Resistance to Immunotherapy in Cancer Patients via Activation of the Macrophage Histamine Receptor H1 (Which was reversed by Antihistamines)

Li, Hongzhong et al.

H1-Antihistamine Treatment Enhances Immunotherapy Response

Summary

"Retrospective analyses revealed that cancer **patients who took antihistamines during immunotherapy treatment had significantly improved survival.** The research team uncovered that histamine and histamine receptor H1 (HRH1) are frequently increased in the tumor microenvironment and induce T cell dysfunction...HRH1 knockout or antihistamine treatment **reverted macrophage immunosuppression, revitalized T cell cytotoxic function, and restored immunotherapy response... Importantly, cancer patients with low plasma histamine levels had a more than *tripled* objective response rate to anti-PD-1 treatment compared with patients with high plasma histamine.** These discoveries warrant prospectively exploring antihistamines as adjuvant agents for combinatorial immunotherapy."

CHAPTER SEVENTEEN

Some Plant-Based PHYTOCHEMICALS are Capable of Blocking or Modulating the PD-1/PD-L1 Signal, Thereby, Enhancing Immunotherapy Efficacy

Incredibly, certain phytochemicals are capable of modulating, blocking, and inhibiting the binding of checkpoints PD-1 to PD-L1. Phytochemicals can be a type of checkpoint inhibitor, exposing previously hidden cancer cells to the immune system, to find, destroy, and remember them for future destruction, thereby enhancing Immunotherapy.

Phytochemicals are plant-based bioactive compounds that occur naturally in vegetables, fruits, whole grains, nuts, seeds, beans, and other legumes.

Phytochemicals can also positively influence the gut microbiome by promoting beneficial bacteria and acting as prebiotics to create a food source for beneficial microbes and can enhance immunotherapy. One of the major classes of phytochemicals is polyphenols, shown below. It is found in fruits, vegetables, herbs, spices, tea, dark chocolate, and wine. Classes of polyphenols include phenolic acids, flavonoids, stilbenes, and lignans.

POLYPHENOLS DIET INFOGRAPHIC

Polyphenols are a group of naturally occurring compounds widely distributed in plants. They feature multiple phenolic rings, which are chemical structures consisting of a six-carbon aromatic ring with a hydroxyl (-OH) group attached. Polyphenols are classified into various subclasses, including flavonoids, phenolic acids, stilbenes, and lignans. Flavonoids are the largest and most studied subclass of polyphenols and are found in high amounts in fruits, vegetables, tea, cocoa, and wine. Polyphenols are known for their antioxidant properties and are responsible for many vibrant colours in fruits, vegetables, and other plant-based foods. Polyphenols are renowned for their health benefits. As potent antioxidants, they can neutralize harmful free radicals in the body, thereby protecting cells and tissues from oxidative damage. They associate with many positive effects on human health. Some polyphenols also possess antimicrobial properties and may contribute to gut health by acting as prebiotics, promoting the growth of beneficial bacteria.

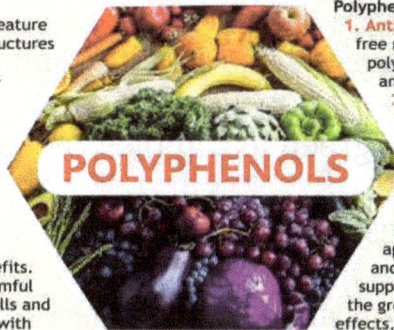

POLYPHENOLS

Polyphenols support health in several ways:
1. **Antioxidant activity:** they can neutralize harmful free radicals in the body. By scavenging free radicals, polyphenols help protect cells from oxidative stress and reduce the risk of oxidative damage.
2. **Anti-inflammatory effects:** help reduce inflammation in the body by suppressing inflammatory processes. 3. **Cardiovascular health:** help lower blood pressure, reduce LDL (bad) cholesterol levels, improve blood vessel function, and inhibit the formation of blood clots. 4. **Anti-cancer activity:** can interfere with cancer cell growth, induce apoptosis (programmed cell death) in cancer cells, and inhibit the formation of new blood vessels that support tumor growth. 5. **Digestive health:** promote the growth of beneficial gut bacteria, provide prebiotic effects, and help maintain a healthy gut microbiota.
6. **Neuroprotective effects:** help protect against age-related cognitive decline and neurodegenerative diseases (such as Alzheimer's and Parkinson's), and improve brain function.

FRUITS
APPLES · BLACK PLUMS · BLACKBERRIES · BLUEBERRIES · CITRUS FRUIT · CRANBERRIES
ELDERBERRIES · POMEGRANATES · RASPBERRIES · RED GRAPES · STRAWBERRIES · TART CHERRIES

VEGETABLES
ARTICHOKES · BEETS · BROCCOLI · BRUSSELS SPROUTS · CARROTS · EGGPLANT
GARLIC · GREEN PEAS · KALE · PEPPERS · PURPLE POTATOES · RADISHES
RED CABBAGE · RED ONIONS · SPINACH · SWEET POTATO · TOMATOES · ZUCCHINI

RED & PURPLE GRAINS
BLACK RICE · PURPLE BARLEY · PURPLE BUCKWHEAT · PURPLE CORN · PURPLE MILLET · PURPLE OATS
PURPLE TEFF · RED AMARANTH · RED QUINOA · RED RICE · RED SORGHUM · RED WHEAT

NUTS AND SEEDS
ALMONDS · CHIA SEEDS · FLAXSEEDS · HAZELNUTS · PECANS · PISTACHIOS · PUMPKIN SEEDS · SESAME SEEDS · SUNFLOWER SEEDS · WALNUTS

HERBS AND SPICES
ALLSPICE · BASIL · BAY LEAVES · BLACK PEPPER · CARDAMOM · CINNAMON · CLOVE BASIL · CLOVES · DILL · GINGER · MARJORAM · NUTMEG · OREGANO · PEPPERMINT · ROSEMARY · SAGE · SAFFRON · TARRAGON · THYME · TURMERIC

OTHER FOODS
BLACK TEA · GREEN TEA · RED WINE · COFFEE · COCOA POWDER · DARK CHOCOLATE · OLIVE OIL

Plant variety, maturity and ripeness, growing conditions, processing and storage, extraction and preparation methods, cooking methods, and food combinations impact polyphenol levels. To maximize polyphenol intake, consuming a diverse range of fruits, vegetables, whole grains, herbs, and spices in their fresh or minimally processed forms is advisable.

This chart is for information only. Always consult a professional before making dietary changes.
dietreminders.com

Classifications of Phytochemicals (Phytonutrients)

Flavonoids are a class of polyphenols that give plants their vibrant colors. They are produced in green tea, red wine, and dark chocolate, broccoli, celery, berries, grapes, carrots, green tea, apples, apricots, leafy greens, nuts, tomatoes, yams, sweet potatoes, onions, cantaloupe, grains, and cereals.

Flavonols are Pale yellow and include Quercetin and myricetin are prominent flavonols.

Anthocyanidins: Produced by red and purple foods such as raspberries, bilberry fruit, and eggplant

Beta-Carotene: Found in orange, yellow vegetables, such as carrots, sweet potatoes, yams, bell peppers, butternut squash, cantaloupe, papaya

Carotenoids, produced in pumpkin, carrots, and red bell peppers,

Catechins, present in black grapes, apricots, and strawberries.

Curcuminoids, contained in turmeric. They are the active plant pigments that are responsible for giving turmeric its bright orange color.

Isoflavones, A type of phytoestrogen produced in soy products, tofu, edamame, miso, tempeh, soybeans, and other legumes such a chickpeas, lentils, split peas, pinto beans, lima beans, and pumpkin seeds.

SOURCES OF PHYTOCHEMICALS

COLOR OF FRUIT AND VEGETABLE GROUPS	SOURCES OF ONE OR MORE OF THE FOLLOWING	FOUND IN ONE OR MORE OF THE FOLLOWING FOODS
GREEN		
	Lutein, Zeaxanthin, Indoles, Vitamin K &/Or Potassium	Turnip, Collard, Kale, Spinach, Lettuce, Broccoli, Green peas, Kiwi, Honeydew, Cabbage, Brussels Sprouts, Bok Choy, Arugala, Swiss Chard, Cauliflower, Leafy greens, Watercress, Endive
YELLOW/ORANGE		
	Beta-Carotene,	Carrots, Sweet potatoes, Pumpkin, Butternut
	Vitamin A, Bioflavonoids, Vitamin C, &/Or Potassium	Squash, Cantaloupe, Mangoes, Apricots, Peaches, Oranges, Grapefruit, Lemons, Tangerines, Clementines, Peaches, Papaya, Nectarines, Pears, Pineapple, Yellow Raisins, Yellow Pepper, Bananas
RED		
	Vitamin C &/Or Anthocyanins	Cranberries, Pink grapefruit, Raspberries, Strawberries, Watermelon, Red Cabbage, Red Pepper, Radishes, Tomatoes, Cherries, Beets, Apples, Red Onion, Kidney Beans, Red Beans
BLUE/PURPLE		
	Anthocyanins, Vitamin C, &/Or Phenolics	Blueberries, Blackberries, Purple Grapes, Black Currants, Elderberries, Plums, Prunes, Raisins, Eggplant
WHITE		
	Allium & Allicin	Garlic, Onions, Leeks, Scallions, Chives

The Immunotherapy Miracle!

Source:

Journal of Cancer

2023 Jul 24;14(12):2315–2328. doi: 10.7150/jca.85966

Combined Use of Immune Checkpoint Inhibitors and Phytochemicals as a Novel Therapeutic Strategy against Cancer

Luo L, Lin C, Wang P, Cao D, Lin Y, Wang W, Zhao Y, Shi Y, Gao Z, Kang X, Zhang Y, Wang S, Wang J, Xu M, Liu H, Liu SL. Combined Use of Immune Checkpoint Inhibitors and Phytochemicals as a Novel Therapeutic Strategy against Cancer. J Cancer. 2023 Jul 24;14(12):2315-2328. doi: 10.7150/jca.85966. PMID: 37576404; PMCID: PMC10414047.

https://pmc.ncbi.nlm.nih.gov/articles/PMC10414047/#ack1. Footnotes are at the site.

"Phyto" means "related to plants." Phytochemicals (also called phytonutrients) are naturally occurring compounds found in plants.

Blocking a PD-1 /PD-L1 Inhibitor, (known as a PD-L1 BLOCKADE) results in the reactivation of the T-cells, allowing them to effectively target and kill the cancer cells by removing the "brake" signal that normally prevents the immune system from attacking cancerous tumor cells.

In substance, it enhances the body's natural anti-tumor immune response by preventing cancer cells from hiding from the immune system. The following Summary shows how most phytochemicals participate in tumor suppression by inhibiting tumor metastasis, angiogenesis, inducing tumor cell apoptosis, and cell cycle arrest.

In pertinent summary, "Phytochemicals enhance immune checkpoint inhibitor therapy *via:*

(A) **Activating immune cells** that recognize and kill cancer cells, such as T cells, Natural Killer (NK) cells, and Dendritic (DC) Cells, as well as suppressing the pro-inflammatory and carcinogenic function of immunosuppressive cells.

(B) **Phytochemicals block the interaction between PD-1 and PD-L1** by decreasing the expression and promoting dimerization/glycosylation of PD-L1, even facilitating their degradation.

(C), Through blocking various cancer signaling pathways such as PI3K/AKT/mTOR, JAK/STAT3, and VEGF. Phytochemicals help Immune Checkpoint Inhibitors to inhibit tumor proliferation, metastasis, and angiogenesis, then induce apoptosis (cancer cell death).

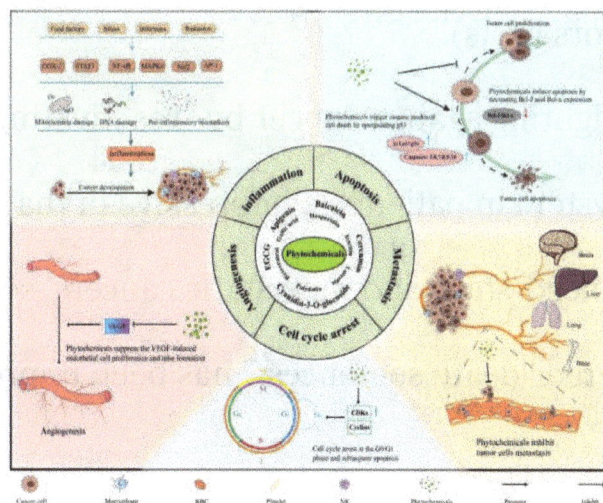

Phytochemicals in Cancer Immune Checkpoint Inhibitor Therapy

Lee J, Han Y, Wang W, Jo H, Kim H, Kim S, Yang KM, Kim SJ, Dhanasekaran DN, Song YS. Phytochemicals in Cancer Immune Checkpoint Inhibitor Therapy. Biomolecules. 2021 Jul 27;11(8):1107. doi: 10.3390/biom11081107. PMID: 34439774; PMCID: PMC8393583. FOOTNOTES TO THE ORIGINAL RESEARCH CAN BE FOUND AT THIS CITE.

Recently, several phytochemicals have been reported to show the modulatory effects of immune checkpoints in various cancers *in vivo* or *in vitro* models. In addition, phytochemicals are capable of suppressing PD-1/PD-L1 binding.

Currently, there has been an increasing interest in cancer immunotherapy, which stimulates the anti-cancer immune system to eliminate malignancy.

To restore the suppressed ability of immune cells to recognize cancer cells, monoclonal antibodies (mAbs) have been adopted as immune checkpoint inhibitors (ICIs).

The idea of fighting against cancer by "reactivating" cancer-inactivated natural immune system in patients is impressive in that the survival rate of patients with advanced-stage and metastatic cancers, some of which, previously considered "death sentences," has been improved dramatically.

What Are Phytochemicals

Phytochemicals are bioactive compounds that occur naturally in vegetables, fruits, whole grains, nuts, seeds, beans, other legumes, and other plant sources. They are essential for protecting plants from insects, microorganisms, and harm caused by bacteria, viruses, and fungi.

Traditional use and continuous observation have demonstrated that extracts from certain plants have therapeutic and preventive effects on various human diseases, a practice known as phytotherapy.

Phytotherapy is a medical science that utilizes plant extracts or phytochemicals to treat diseases or enhance overall health. The natural compounds contained in plant extracts exhibit a wide range of biological activities in the human body, including antioxidation, immune-boosting, anti-inflammatory effects, and cardiovascular health maintenance. These are not vitamins or minerals, but they offer significant healing benefits. In addition to being PD-1/PD-L1 modulators and blockers, phytochemicals are capable of stopping genetic damage or otherwise interfering with the initiation, promotion, and progression of cancer.

A substantial body of evidence also supports the effectiveness of phytochemicals in preventing and treating various diseases.

In addition to cancer, these include cardiovascular disease, strokes, neurological conditions, diabetes, osteoporosis, cataracts, menopausal conditions, gastroenteric disorders, atopic eczema, hyperactivity, and gynecological issues.

Phytonutrients also positively influence the gut microbiome by promoting beneficial bacteria and acting as prebiotics to feed the microbiome.

Phytochemicals Shown in Clinical Trials to Modulate, Block and Inhibit PD-1 / PD-L1 to Enhance Immunotherapy and Unleash the Immune System Against Cancer

Certain phytochemicals have been shown in Clinical Studies to be capable of creating immune-stimulating checkpoint blocks and modulations to the PD1/PD-L1 signal to enhance immunotherapy and unleash the immune system to destroy cancer cells.

These phytonutrients include anthocyanins, lycopene, capsaicinoids, ginsenoside, diosgenin, sulforaphane, quercetin, baicalin, silymarin, apigenin, luteolin, carotin, EGCG: epigallocatechin gallate, C3G: Cyanidin 3-*O*-glucoside; CAPE: caffeic acid, phenethyls, resveratrol, curcumin, and other studied phytochemicals.

PD-1/PD-L1 Modulators and Blockers FOOD SOURCES

Anthocyanins are a powerhouse of phytonutrients, found primarily in purple and blue foods such as red and purple grapes, blueberries, blackberries, raspberries, cranberries, acai berries, cherries, pomegranates, and plums; as well as vegetables such as purple eggplant, red potatoes, and purple cabbage.

EGCG, a catechin found in green tea.

Luteolin, found in broccoli, carrots, cabbage, and rosemary;

Silymarin, also known as milk thistle, is a liver detoxifier. It is found in milk thistle and artichokes.

Hesperidin. Abundant in the fruit and peels of citrus fruits such as lemons, limes, oranges, and grapefruit, as well as kiwifruit, onions, and garlic.

Curcumin. Curcumin is the main active compound in turmeric. It is a potent anti-inflammatory and is in curry powder. Ginger is a member of the same family as curcumin. Cayenne pepper may also provide curcumin.

Gallic Acid. A naturally occurring polyphenol found in green tea, grapes, strawberries, blueberries, blackberries, raspberries, black currants, plums, cherries, pomegranates, walnuts, cashews, and hazelnuts.

Polydatin – (Also called **picid**). Found in blueberries and cranberries and grapes, and foods with resveratrol. It is also in peanuts, pistachios, and cocoa products. Polydatin is also found in hops cones used in beer brewing.

Resveratrol. A powerful polyphenol found in red wine is concentrated in the skins and seeds of grapes and berries. It is abundant in blueberries, cranberries, and other berries (fresh or frozen). It is also found in peanuts, pistachios, cocoa, and dark chocolate.

Berberine: Barberry fruit.

Piceatannol. Found in passion fruit, black grapes, blueberries, peanuts, almonds, and white tea in lesser amounts than resveratrol,

Emodin. Most notably found in rhubarb, also in buckthorn, knotweed, senna, aloe vera, peas, and cabbage,

CAPE. Honey, spices such as cloves and herbs such as oregano, rosemary, and mint, as well as cranberries, blueberries, and strawberries..

Terpenes

Lycopene. Carotenoid pigment is found in red, pink, and orange fruits and vegetables such as Tomatoes, watermelon, pink grapefruit, papaya, persimmons, and apricots. Lycopene is also found in red bell peppers, carrots, sweet potatoes, tomato sauce, and ketchup also contain lycopene.

Saponins. Widely found in legumes, oats, quinoa, amaranth, soybeans, chickpeas, lentils, navy beans, kidney beans, yams, spinach, asparagus, millet, tea leaves, and coffee.

CHAPTER EIGHTEEN

Mechanisms of Phytochemicals Shown to Modulate or Block the PD-1/PD-L1 Pathway

The following phytochemicals have been shown in clinical trials to be capable of blocking or modulating the PD-1/PD-L1 signal to enhance Checkpoint Inhibitor Immunotherapy to UNLEASH the immune system against cancer cells.

The ELISA Assay

In most cases, this PD-1/PD-L1 modulating or blocking ability is determined by an ELISA Assay (Enzyme-Linked Immunosorbent Assay).

ELISA is a widely used laboratory technique that is used to detect and quantify the binding of PD-1 to PD-L1, with, in the case of these studies, a particular phytochemical, relying on the highly specific binding between an antibody and its corresponding antigen.

Anthocyanins

Anthocyanins are a powerhouse of phytonutrients, found primarily in purple and blue foods such as blueberries, bilberries, blackberries, raspberries, cranberries, grapes, cherries, pomegranates, and plums; as well as vegetables such as purple eggplant, red potatoes, and purple cabbage.

The Immunotherapy Miracle!

Anthocyanins and their metabolites can significantly inhibit the expression of both PD-1 and PD-L1, stimulating an immune response and suppressing cancer progression. Additionally, a study on the microbiome revealed the connection between the intestinal flora alteration by anthocyanins.

It was also reported that the efficacy of anti-PD-1 or anti-PD-L1 monoclonal antibodies can be increased with the oral supplement of *Akkermansia muciniphila*, a beneficial strain of probiotic bacteria.

This probiotic lives on the mucus lining of the gut. The prebiotic foods that this power probiotic prefers are pomegranate, raspberries, blueberries, blackberries, cranberries, grapes, apples, walnuts, pecans, and green tea, which are primarily anthocyanins.

Research shows that "patients with this gut bacteria are more likely to respond to cancer treatment and stimulate their immune system to kill cancer.

In clinical studies, this compositional alteration in the gut microbiome boosted the production of anti-cancer and anti-inflammatory short-chain fatty acids, especially butyrate, which impacts inflammation and immune function. It has also been shown to impact mental health. Anthocyanins also enhance intertumoral CD8+ Killer T cell infiltration.

C3G (*Cyanidin-3-O-glucoside):*

According to science researchers (Candice Mazewski et al. Sci Rep 2019), C3G has the possibility of a non-drug treatment that inhibits PD1/ PD-L1 expression. C3G significantly inhibited PD-L1 in colon cancer cell lines. By inhibiting PD-L1 expression, C3G may enhance the effectiveness of immunotherapy checkpoint inhibitors. C3G is the major type of anthocyanin and is a pigment responsible for the red, purple, and blue colors in fruits and vegetables, including pomegranates, blackberries, bilberries, elderberries, mulberries, as well as black rice, black beans, and purple potatoes.

Apigenin

Apigenin-rich foods include celery, parsley, onions, rutabagas, artichokes, cilantro, oranges, spinach, tea, thyme, and hot peppers.

Coombs et al. (Cancer Lett. 2016; 380:424–433. doi: 10.1016) showed that apigenin inhibited PD-L1 expression in human and mouse breast cancer cells. Apigenin is a flavone (a class of flavonoid) abundantly present in fruits and vegetables. Apigenin has been shown to reduce PD-L1 levels in various cancer cell types, including melanoma and breast cancer cells.

This inhibition of PD-L1 expression can potentially enhance anti-tumor responses by reducing the *suppression* of T cells against cancer cells.

The benefits of apigenin include free-radical scavenging, antimicrobial activity, suppression of cancer cell growth, and anti-inflammatory effects. Similar results have been reported in melanoma studies. When melanoma cells were treated with apigenin or curcumin, PD-L1 was remarkably suppressed. Additionally, treatment with apigenin or curcumin in melanoma-bearing mice significantly suppressed tumor growth by inhibiting PD-L1 expression in melanoma cells. Compared to curcumin, apigenin led to greater suppressive activity. Inflammation-induced PD-L1 can also be inhibited by apigenin.

Luteolin

In clinical studies, it has been shown that luteolin, the metabolite of apigenin, inhibits the expression of PD-L1.

Luteolin was also shown to inhibit several signaling pathways that were necessary for cancer cell survival.

The disruption of the interaction between PD-1 and PD-L1, immune checkpoint inhibitors can restore immune system function against cancer cells, resulting in their destruction. Growing evidence has demonstrated that, with their potent anti-inflammatory, antioxidant, and anticancer properties, apigenin and luteolin induce apoptosis (cancer cell destruction) in multiple types of cancer cells.

In the case study, ZB Jiang (2021) luteolin and apigenin significantly inhibited lung cancer cell growth and induced apoptosis, initiated cell cycle arrest, decreased angiogenesis and stopped metastasis, and reduced cell proliferation.

Good sources of luteolin include celery, parsley, broccoli, green bell peppers, onions, and citrus fruits. Luteolin is also found in herbs such as Sage, Rosemary, and Thyme. Additionally, spinach, apples, capers, and green tea are good sources.

Astaxanthin

Astaxanthin is a carotenoid and a powerful antioxidant that plays a role in the inactivation of PD-1 sites on T-cells and the activation of Natural Killer Cells.

Astaxanthin also corrects intracellular, extracellular, and membrane concentrations of the abnormal electrical properties of cancer cells, which includes a reduction of PD-L1 and PD-1 activity, resulting in stimulating the immune system to destroy cancer cells.

Astaxanthin, further, gives cancer cells more oxidative stress that inhibits their growth.

Astragaloside IV (Astragalus Root)

Astragaloside IV, a key component of astragalus, has been shown to modulate PD-L1 molecules and Immune Checkpoint Inhibitors.

Astragalus has been widely used in traditional Chinese medicine for the treatment of viral and bacterial infections, inflammation, as well as cancer.

Its medicinal properties are concentrated in the Astragalus root. It is not in foods, so it is typically taken in supplement form. The root can also be used to make tea. Astragalus contains cycloastragenol (CAG), which can act as a telomerase activator to prevent the destruction of telomeres, which are markers on your DNA that cause you to age as they shorten.

In cancer, it has been shown to inhibit cell proliferation, promote cell apoptosis, inhibit metastasis, inhibit angiogenesis, and enhance immunity.

Recently, scientific researchers Liu, Chen, and Wang (2021) found that astragaloside IV inhibits epithelial-mesenchymal transition (EMT) (which is linked to cancer cell invasion, metastasis, and stem cell properties). It also inhibits angiogenesis (growth of new blood vessels) in gastric cancer.

Meng et al. (2020) reported that astragaloside IV enhanced the inhibition of the PD-1 monoclonal antibody in lung cancer.
Astragalus polysaccharide (APS) has an inhibitory effect on a variety of solid cancer tumors, which is related to the up-regulation of PD-L1.

Baicalein (Baicalin)

Baicalein and its conjugate baicalin, are a flavonoids found in skull cap roots. Ke et al. found that baicalein and baicalin significantly inhibited tumor growth and immunosuppression by regulating PD-L1 expression in liver cancer cells. The inhibition of STAT3 (a transcriptional factor involved in almost all features of cancer), by baicalein and baicalin, suppressed IFN-γ (interferon gamma) -induced PD-L1 expression and increased T cell-mediated liver cancer cell death. This suggests the possibility of inhibiting the immune evasion of cancer cells. It has a role as an antioxidant, an angiogenic agent, a hormone antagonist, and an anti-inflammatory agent. Many research studies suggest that baicalein and baicalin have antitumor effects, such as cancer cell apoptosis. It is not found in food but is in thyme and can be taken in supplement form.

Caffeic Acid Phenethyl Ester (CAPE)

Caffeic acid phenethyl ester (CAPE), a hydroxycinnamic acid, is a class of phenolic acids that has been shown to have immunomodulatory effects, potentially influencing the tumor microenvironment and impacting the effectiveness of therapies targeting the PD-1/PD-L1 pathways. It also has potential antioxidant and anti-inflammatory effects.

CAPE is an important active component of honeybee propolis extract. Foods that contain CAPE include honey, brewed coffee, red wine, black choke berries, olives, cabbage, artichokes, dried fruits, prunes, apple sauce, cranberries, blueberries, and strawberries, sunflower seeds, and herbs such as basil, sage, cloves, oregano, rosemary, and mint.

CAPE is a major polyphenol responsible for maintaining normal levels of nitric oxide. Nitric oxide (NO) is a crucial signaling molecule that relaxes and widens blood vessels, which increases blood flow and regulates blood pressure. It also helps deliver oxygen and nutrients to the body's tissues, which improves circulation and endurance and helps eliminate blood clots.

Curcumin

Curcumin is a non-flavonoid polyphenolic compound that can modulate the PD-1/PD-L1 pathway and enhance the effectiveness of immunotherapy and anti-tumor immunity. By reducing PD-L1, curcumin can make it harder for cancer cells to suppress T-cells. This can lead to increased T-Cell activity and potentially better tumor killing. Research suggests that curcumin can be used in combination with traditional PD-1/PD-L1 checkpoint inhibitors to enhance results.

Curcumin is the primary active compound in turmeric and is a potent anti-inflammatory agent. It is present in curry powder, which is in the ginger family. Cayenne pepper may also contain small amounts of curcumin.

Recent studies have reported that curcumin may be a potential agent for improving the response of immunotherapy.

Curcumin also improves the function of CD8+ T cells (killer T cells), which are crucial for attacking cancer cells, leading to a more effective anti-tumor response.

Diosgenin

Diosgenin is a steroidal saponin. Diosgenin does not directly block PD-1 but is an antitumor compound that enhances the efficacy of anti-PD-1 monoclonal antibodies.

Diosgenin is a natural steroid precursor that occurs naturally in certain plants, such as fenugreek seeds and the roots of wild yams (not to be confused with the sweet potato yam). Diosgenin is the precursor in the production of synthetic sterol hormones like progesterone and cortisol. For this reason, it is not recommended to be taken by someone with hormone-receptor-positive breast cancer. It has shown potential against liver, lung, prostate, pancreatic, esophageal, and cervical cancers.

Diosgenin can be found in wild yams, fenugreek, carrots, wild carrots, and bitter gourd. It is anti-inflammatory, immune-modulating, lipid-lowering, antiviral, and anticancer. In melanoma, diosgenin suppressed cell viability and promoted apoptosis (programmed cell death) and inhibited metastasis. The combined administration of anti-PD-1 monoclonal antibody with diosgenin generated tumor apoptosis by eliciting augmented T-cell responses (Dong, Meng, et al., 2018, Diosgenin promotes antitumor immunity and PD-1 efficacy against melanoma by regulating intestinal microbiota).

EGCG, Green Tea Extract

Epigallocatechin gallate (EGCG), the most abundant catechin found in green tea, is a potent antioxidant flavan-3-ol (subclass of flavonol) with proven anti-cancer effects in multiple cancer studies. (Rawangkan et al. Rawangkan A, Wongsirisin P, Namiki K, Iida K, Kobayashi Y, Shimizu Y, Fujiki H, Suganuma M. *Green Tea Catechin as an Alternative Immune Checkpoint Inhibitor that Inhibits PD-L1 Expression and Lung Tumor Growth.*)

Molecules, 2018 Aug 18;23(8):2071) demonstrated that EGCG and green tea extract suppressed PD-L1 expression in Non-Small Cell Lung Cancer cells, induced by interferon gamma (IFN-γ) and Epidermal Growth Factor (EGF). Using a mouse model, oral administration of 14% EGCG green tea extract significantly reduced PD-L1-positive cells of lung tumors.

Furthermore, the PD-L1 suppressing effect of EGCG was also evaluated in mouse melanoma cells using a T cell co-culture experiment. Compared with melanoma cells only, EGCG highly reduced PD-L1 mRNA expression in T cell co-cultured melanoma cells. EGCG also increased the number of T cells, indicating the restoration of T cell activity by PD-L1 inhibition. Further studies on EGCG with PD-1/PD-L1 inhibitors may significantly increase the Immune Checkpoint Inhibiting therapeutic effect.

Both green tea and Matcha come from the same plant, *Camellia sinensis,* but Matcha powder contains a significantly greater amount of EGCG than green tea.

Although the amount can vary, according to the USDA National Nutritional Data Base, a typical serving of 1 gram of Matcha contains about 30-40 mg of EGCG.

In comparison, regular green tea typically contains around. 10-20 mg of EGCG per cup

A few weeks before harvest, the tea leaves are shielded from sunlight. This increases the amount of theanine, an amino acid that contributes to matcha's unique umami flavor.

Matcha is made by consuming the entire green tea leaf in powdered form. It has a higher nutrient content than green tea.

Because black tea and Oolong teas are fermented, which requires converting catechins to tannins, there are fewer catechins in these teas compared to Matcha.

Emodin.

Emodin is an anthraquinone most notably found in rhubarb. It is also found in buckthorn, knotweed, senna, aloe vera, peas, and cabbage.

Emodin has been shown to attenuate PD-L1 stabilization, resulting in decreased PD-L1 binding and enhanced T-cell-mediated tumor cell death.

It has promising effects in cancer research due to its anti-cancer properties. Emodin is effective against a wide range of cancer types, including lung, breast, liver, and pancreatic cancer.

It works by inducing apoptosis, inhibiting cell proliferation and growth, and suppressing cell invasion and metastasis.

Fisetin

Studies indicate that fisetin has been shown to block the interaction between PD-1 and PD-L1 in competitive ELISA assays. This makes fisetin a potential candidate for use as an immune checkpoint inhibitor.

The powerhouse, Fisetin, is found in strawberries, onions, grapes, mangoes, apples, persimmons, cruciferous vegetables such as broccoli, leafy greens, tomatoes, cucumbers, fatty fish, ginger, turmeric, and dark chocolate.

Gallic Acid.

A naturally occurring polyphenol found in green tea, grapes, strawberries, blueberries, blackberries, raspberries, black currants, plums, and cherries.

Studies suggest that Gallic acid can indirectly influence the PD-1 / PD-L1 signaling pathway by reducing the expression levels of PD-L1. Gallic acid can also affect the regulatory T cells (Treg Cells), which are cells that can suppress the anti-tumor response and enhance the attack to destroy the cancer tumor.

Combining gallic acid with an anti-PD-1 monoclonal antibody may lead to a greater anti-tumor effect than using either alone. It can enhance the effectiveness of the PD-1 blockade to unleash the immune system.

Ginger. Some clinical studies suggest that ginger and the compound 6-gingerol can potentially block PD-1 and PD-L1 signaling interactions and enhance immune responses against cancer, through ginger's anti-inflammatory and anticancer properties. ("Anticancer Effects of 6-Gingerol through downregulating Iron Transport and PD-L1 Expression in Non-Small Cell Lung Cancer Cells" (Kang, Park, et al. Nov. 15, 2023).

Ginger is cooked into a variety of foods such as curries, stir-fried, soups, stews, marinades, and sauces. It's in baked goods such as ginger snaps and drinks such as ginger ale. It's also served pickled.

Hesperidin

Hesperidin is a flavone in the class of flavonoids. It is abundant in fruit and peels of citrus fruits such as lemons, limes, oranges, and grapefruit. It is also contained in kiwifruit, onions, and garlic. Hesperidin has anti-cancer effects in several types of cancer. In triple-negative breast cancer, it was shown that, in cell lines that highly expressed PD-L1, hesperidin downregulated PD-L1 expression.

This was achieved by suppressing Akt, which is a critical signaling pathway that plays a major role in cancer development and progression, and the NF-kb pathway, involved in various cellular processes, particularly inflammation and immune responses. This indicates the potential role of hesperidin as an Immune Checkpoint Inhibitor drug.

Icaritin

Icaritin is not found in food. It is a flavonoid obtained from the *Epimedium genus* plant, also known as 'horny goat Weed," and it is used in traditional Chinese medicine for its tonic and stamina-boosting properties.

The anti-cancer effects of icaritin, such as cancer cell growth inhibition and apoptosis, have been studied in various cancers, including hepatocellular carcinoma, glioblastoma, ovarian cancer, and cervical cancer.

Mo, Zhu, Wang, et al. (Icaritin inhibits PD-L1 expression by targeting Protein IkB Kinase) showed the possibility of icaritin as an immune therapeutic agent in liver cancer. Icaritin reduced cancer cell proliferation and was also shown to suppress PD-L1 expression.

Icaritin also inhibited the translocation of NF-κB p65, which acts on the promoter of PD-L1.

Therefore, icaritin, which exhibits immunomodulatory activities in various carcinomas, can regulate immune checkpoint expression and has great potential for adjuvant treatment with Immunotherapy Checkpoint Inhibitor therapy.

Kaempferol

Kaempferol is a type of flavanol that has also been shown to inhibit the interaction between PD-1 and PD-L1, making it a potential PD-L1 blocker with the power to unleash the immune system against cancer cells. Foods high in kaempferol include apples, grapes, pomegranate, kale, broccoli, cauliflower, radishes, brussels sprouts, spinach, onions, and garlic. Kaempferol is also contained in citrus fruits.

Lycopene

A Carotenoid pigment found in red, pink, and orange fruits and vegetables, such as Tomatoes, watermelon, pink grapefruit, papaya, persimmons, and apricots. Lycopene is also found in red bell peppers, carrots, and sweet potatoes. Processed tomato products such as tomato sauce, catsup, and other tomato products.

Lycopene has been shown to synergistically improve the efficacy of anti-PD-1 therapy by reducing PD-L1 expression and boosting immune response.

Myricetin. The flavonoid Myricetin is structurally similar and has many of the same functions as the flavonols, fisetin, luteolin, and quercetin. It can be produced from kaempferol, another flavanol.

Myricetin has been shown in Clinical Studies to inhibit interferon-γ-induced PD-L1 expression in certain cancer cell types, such as lung cancer cells. This suggests that it might have the potential to inhibit the PD-1/PD-L1 checkpoint signal and ignite the immune system against cancer. It is particularly abundant in berries, such as cranberries, blueberries, strawberries, goji berries, black currants, and bilberries. It is also found in nuts and carrots, and fennel leaves, as well as leafy greens such as chard.

Other sources include kale, broccoli, brussels sprouts, and cabbage. Carrots, turnips, and peas, as well as buckwheat and capers. This flavonoid is also found in oranges and apples, as well as nuts, tea, and red wine.

Naringenin

Naringenin belongs to the flavanone group of polyphenols and is found mainly in citrus fruits like grapefruits and others, such as tomatoes and cherries. Naringenin can block the interaction between PD-1 and PD-L1 according to research published by the National Institute of Health (NIH). This blockage is a key mechanism for immunotherapy checkpoint inhibitors in cancer therapy. Naringenin has also been shown to activate T cells in co-culture systems, suggesting its potential as a natural blocker for PD-1/PD-L1 interactions. Available evidence demonstrates that <u>naringenin</u> has important pharmacological properties, including anti-inflammatory, antioxidant, <u>neuroprotective</u>, hepatoprotective, and anti-cancer activities.

Collected data shows the inactivation of carcinogens after treatment with pure naringenin and naringenin-loaded <u>nanoparticles</u> in various malignancies, such as colon cancer, lung neoplasms, breast cancer, leukemia and lymphoma, pancreatic cancer, prostate tumors, oral squamous cell carcinoma, liver cancer, brain tumors, skin cancer, cervical, ovarian cancer, bladder neoplasms, gastric cancer, and osteosarcoma.

Naringenin inhibits cancer progression through multiple mechanisms, like apoptosis induction, cell cycle arrest, angiogenesis hindrance, and modification of various signaling pathways.

Olive Leaf Extract and Oleuropein

Olive Leaf extract and the phenolic compound oleuropein, a compound found in olive leaves, **can enhance the effectiveness of PD-1 Immunotherapy**. It has been shown to potentiate the PD-1 blockade and decrease PD-L1 levels in some cancer models.

It is believed that oleuropein influences the immune system in ways that enhance T-Cell immune responses and make the tumor more vulnerable to the PD-1 blockade. This suggests that olive leaf extract might help boost the effectiveness of PD1/PD-L1 therapies. It has also been shown to inhibit the growth of cancer cells and to inhibit the spread of metastatic melanoma.

Silymarin - (Silibinin as its key constituent)

Silymarin is a complex of flavonolignans extracted from the plant milk thistle (*Silybum marianum*), commonly used for liver disease treatment.

It has been shown to suppress P-L1 and cancer cell proliferation in colorectal cancer cells and increase Killer T-Cells in tumor-bearing mice.

Silybin is the main bioactive flavonolignan of silymarin, proven to inhibit STAT3 signaling in many types of cancer cells.

Several studies indicated a suppressive effect of silibinin on PD-L1 in cancer cells. (Cuyàs, W., Perez-Sanchez, A., et al., 2016) revealed that silibinin treatment of non-small lung cancer cells significantly reduced the mRNA expression of PD-L1.

It further reduced epithelial-mesenchymal transition (EMT) regulators (which are crucial for increased cancer invasiveness and metastasis) via the inhibition of STAT3 phosphorylation. STAT3 plays a crucial role in cancer development and progression, such as cancer cell growth, proliferation, and survival.

Sulforaphane and Organosulfur Compounds

Organic sulfur compounds can BLOCK the interaction between PD-1 and PD-L1. There are two main kinds of compounds, one is glucosinolate, which are sulfur-containing compound, and its hydrolyzed product isothiocyanate (ITCs) found in cruciferous plants, such as broccoli, cauliflower, brussels sprouts, and cabbage. The other is allyl sulfide.

Allyl sulfide is mainly in Liliaceae Allium, which is especially abundant in garlic, as well as onions, shallots, leeks and chives, and mustard seeds.

Small molecule inhibitors, including those containing organic sulfur, can bind to PD-L1 and prevent it from binding to PD-1, thus interfering with the immune checkpoint pathway that ignites the immune system to kill cancer.

Clinical Trial Results showed that sulforaphane enhanced the cytotoxic (cancer-killing) function and inhibited PD-1, as well as PDL1 expression.

Clinical studies showed that, in lung cancer, the PD-1/PD-L1 inhibition was induced by IFN-γ (interferon-gamma), which is a signaling molecule produced by immune cells such as T cells and natural killer cells. These act as messengers to activate other immune cells to regulate the immune response. Interferon-gamma plays a role in fighting cancer.

Piceatannol.

Another type of phytonutrient is a stilbenoid, which is a natural compound found in passion fruit, black grapes, red wine, blueberries, peanuts, almonds, and white tea in lesser amounts than resveratrol. Piceatannol has been shown to upregulate the PD-L1 expression on cancer cells to enhance the effectiveness of PD-1/PD-L1 checkpoint blockade immunotherapy.

Polydatin

Polydatin is a natural polyphenol and a precursor to Resveratrol. Foods containing polydatin include guava, lemons, grapes, berries, such as blueberries, blackberries, mulberries, and strawberries, as well as peanuts, pistachios, dark chocolate, and red wine. It is also contained in hops cones used in beer brewing. Polydatin, also called *piceid,* can block PD-L1 expression, which helps the immune system to target and destroy cancer cells.

It inhibits PD-L1 by regulating miR-382, a microRNA that specifically targets PD-L1. It has also been shown to have antitumor effects such as apoptosis (cancer suicide) and anti-proliferation of various cancer types, including colorectal cancer.

Resveratrol

Resveratrol (RSV) is a type of natural stilbene polyphenol that suppresses PD-L1 and has been shown to target and block PD-L1 to enhance antitumor T-cell cancer killing ability. Resveratrol is one of the most well-known phytochemicals. It has been reported to have various biological effects, such as antioxidant, free-radical scavenging, cardioprotective, neuroprotective, anti-microbial, and anti-cancer activity.

Resveratrol is found in red wine and is concentrated in the skins and seeds of red and purple grapes and berries. It is abundant in blueberries, blackberries, raspberries, acai berries, cranberries, goji berries, mulberries, and other berries (fresh or frozen). It is also found in peanuts, peanut butter, pistachios, cocoa, and dark chocolate.

Resveratrol also has a regulatory effect on the immune system. It is a polyphenol that can reduce the expression of pro-inflammatory genes, which protects the body against oxidative damage. Resveratrol can also induce anti-proliferation in various cancer cells and inhibit cancer growth in vivo.

Numerous studies have shown that Resveratrol can directly and indirectly control cancer cells and immune cells, enabling the regulation of immune responses in various types of cancer.

Mushrooms

Research indicates that certain compounds derived from mushrooms can act as a PD-1/PD-L1 modulators.

Lentinan and Beta-Glucan

A Polysaccharide derived from the shitake mushroom. It has been shown to downregulate the PD-L1 pathway. It contains beta-glucan, a common mushroom polysaccharide that can act as an immune adjuvant.

It enhances immune cell activity and immune function, which can potentially enhance the effectiveness of PD-1/PD-L1 checkpoint blockade therapies.

Beta Glucan has been shown to inhibit tumor growth and angiogenesis (formation of new blood vessels to the cancer tumor). It can also impact cell regulation and apoptosis. Increase Killer T Cells.

Ganoderma Lucidum

Research on Reishi mushrooms and Ganoderma lucidum found in them indicates that their bioactive compounds can reduce PD-1 protein levels in immune cells, suggesting a role in modulating the PD-1/PD-L1 pathway.

Turkey Tail Mushrooms

These are powerful, cancer-killing mushrooms. They have been shown in clinical studies to act as non-specific immune modulators.

A 2012 study found that breast cancer patients who took turkey tail recovered immune function after radiation. Other research shows that turkey tail mushrooms also have anti-tumor properties. Following is a link for an empowering Ted Talk by Paul Stamets, author and the leading expert on mushrooms, explaining how his mother was cured from Stage IV breast and liver cancer with turkey tail mushrooms. Go to the following website:

https://video.search.yahoo.com/search/video?fr=mcafee&p=Paul+St
amets+turkey+tail+mushroom+Ted+Talk&type=E211US1274G0#id=7
&vid=3e4d58d849628acd238c4cef701c7a4&action

Proanthocyanidins

Proanthocyanidins are found in grape seed extract derived from grape oligomers of monomeric catechins and epicatechins, which are potential cancer-fighting agents due to their antioxidant and anti-inflammatory properties. Research suggests they can inhibit cancer cell growth, induce apoptosis, and potentially prevent metastasis. Grape seed extract has demonstrated these effects in various cancer types, including lung, breast, and colorectal cancers.

Pectin

Pectin is a polysaccharide. It is a type of soluble fiber found naturally on the cell walls of fruits and vegetables, particularly citrus peels and apple pomace, and is used as a gelling agent.

Research suggests that pectin may enhance the effectiveness of anti-PD-1 immunotherapy, which targets the receptor that binds to PD-L1.

Modified citrus pectin has been shown to interact with Galectin-3, a protein implicated in various cancer hallmarks, including immune regulation.

Inhibition of Galectin-3 may contribute to an anti-tumor response. Pectin has also been associated with other immunomodulatory effects, such as reducing inflammation and promoting apoptosis.

Quercetin

Quercetin is one of the most powerful flavanols, shown to inhibit PD-1/PD-L1 interactions. It is a powerful antioxidant that helps stabilize *mast cells,* which release histamine during allergic reactions. It can flush out histamines, enhancing immunotherapy and eliminating certain side effects.

Onions are a particularly rich source of quercetin. It is also found in broccoli, kale, and tomatoes, as well as raspberries, blackberries, blueberries, cranberries, apples, red grapes, capers, citrus fruits, and peanuts.

Source:

Quercetin inhibits the PD-1/PD-L1 interaction for an immune-enhancing cancer chemopreventive agent.

Lei Jing [1,2], Jieru Lin [1], Yang Yang [1], Li Tao [1], Yuyin Li [1], Zhenxing Liu [1], Qing Zhao [1], Aipo Diao [1]

Quercetin inhibits the PD-1/PD-L1 interaction for an immune-enhancing cancer chemopreventive agent. Phytother Res. 2021 Nov;35(11):6441-6451. doi: 10.1002/ptr.7297. Epub 2021 Sep 24. PMID: 34560814.

Quercetin dihydrate was shown to inhibit the PD-1/PD-L1 interaction.

These results suggest that quercetin dihydrate attenuates the inhibitory effect of PD-L1 on T cells by inhibiting the PD-1/PD-L1 interaction, which has the powerful potential to be used as a cancer chemopreventive agent ("a natural compound that prevents, reverses, or blocks cancer").

Targeting the PD-1/PD-L1 immune checkpoints has achieved significantly positive results in the treatment of multiple cancers.

Quercetin is one of the most abundant dietary flavonoids found in various vegetables and fruits and has a wide range of biological activities, including immunomodulation.

Quercetin is widely found in fruits and vegetables (Di Petrillo et al., 2022). Several studies highlight the anti-oxidation, antiviral, antimicrobial, anti-inflammatory, and antitumor properties of quercetin (Davoodvandi et al., 2020; Di Petrillo et al., 2022). This showed strong effects in PD-1/PD-L1 binding suppression and PD-L1 down-regulation.

Studies on Quercetin also showed cytotoxic T cells (killer cells) activation, DCs maturation, and tumor inhibition.

Qiu et al. (2021) elucidated that quercetin downregulated PD-L1 expression, promoted an increase, and synergized cytotoxic effects of γδ (gamma delta T cells with tumor killing capabilities) on breast cancer cells. (These T cells are often found in the epithelial tissues and are thought to play a role in early immune responses, particularly at mucosal surfaces.

The Immunotherapy Miracle!

Expression of PD-L1 on osteosarcoma cells is dramatically decreased under quercetin treatment, due to the inhibition of the JAK2-STAT3 signaling pathway (which plays a vital role in cancer cell growth and immune responses (Jing et al., 2022).

Furthermore, a syngeneic tumor model was established to reveal that **quercetin combined with anti-PD-1 therapy significantly inhibited tumor growth**.

Quercetin dihydrate was found to inhibit the PD-1/ PD-L1 binding, which further stimulates T cell activation and suppresses tumor growth (Jing et al., 2021).

Additionally, Quercetin dihydrate stimulates CD8 (killer T cells), the most powerful effectors in the anticancer immune response and the backbone of current successful cancer immunotherapies, directly killing cancer cells.

Granzyme B, produced by cytotoxic T-cells and NK Cells, plays a crucial role in the immune system's ability to eliminate cancer cells. IFN-γ (interferon gamma) protein levels in tumor tissues were also increased.

Researchers in Italy found that supplementing quercetin (a hydrophobic, fat-soluble nutrient) by complexing it with phospholipids from sunflower oil (a complex known as a "phosphosome") was **20 times better absorbed, resulting in significantly higher blood levels of quercetin**, compared to regular quercetin, which was not bound by a phospholipid. (Riva A. Ronchi, Petrangolini G, et al, Improved Oral Absorption of Quercetin.)

Phytosomes are a Delivery System that Dramatically Increase the Bioavailability of Hydrophobic – (Not dissolvable in Water) Phytochemicals

"Phytosome is a new delivery system based on food-grade lecithin" Eu J Drug Metab Pharmacokinet 2019; 44 (2:169-177). ("Quercetin Phytosome consists of quercetin and sunflower lecithin in a 1:1 weight ratio.")

In a recent review, phytosomes were listed to enhance to bioavailability of phytochemicals from quercetin, curcumin, silymarin, milk thistle, ginkgo biloba, grape seed extract, and green tea (EGCG).

CHAPTER NINETEEN

How to Maximize the Assimilation of Fat-Soluble Phytochemicals and Nutrients into the Body

There is an often quoted statement in the field of Nutrition that "You are what you eat." However, it might be more appropriately stated as. "You are what your body absorbs."

Hydrophobic foods and phytochemicals are fat-soluble and do not dissolve in water. (Hydro means "water" and phobic means "fearing"). Conversely, the suffix "philic" means "having an affinity or an attraction to something." Hydrophilic foods, phytochemicals, nutrients, and vitamins are "water-loving" and can be assimilated in the body with water.

Fat-soluble vitamins include Vitamins A, D, E, and K.

Fat-soluble foods, phytochemicals, vitamins, and nutrients require the addition of lipids (fats) such as fatty foods for maximum absorption.

Fat-soluble phytochemicals include those not soluble in water.

To increase the absorption of fat-soluble phytochemicals such as lycopene, beta-carotene, lutein, zeaxanthin, quercetin, curcumin, resveratrol, polydatin, hesperidin, berberine, and EGCG in green tea or matcha, milk thistle, and ginkgo biloba, you can pair them with healthy fats.

These can include avocado, olive oil, coconut oil, butter, full-fat milk, or yogurt.

Adding black pepper, containing piperine, to curcumin can dramatically increase its bioavailability. Cooking tomatoes can increase lycopene.

Also, supplements with "liposomal-based phytosomes" added to the phytochemical make it significantly more absorbable "bioavailable" to the cells and the body.

Liposomes and Phytosomes

Liposomes and phytosomes are both lipid-based delivery systems for fat-based phytochemicals and nutrients, used to enhance the bioavailability and efficacy of bioactive compounds. However, they differ in structure and how they interact with the active ingredient.

Phytosomes resemble liposomes, but the active phytocomponents are chemically bound to the phospholipid head groups rather than simply encapsulated within a lipid bio-layer. This creates a lipid-compatible molecular structure and improves the solubility and permeability of plant compounds.

Phospholipids are formed by the interaction between plant extracts with phospholipids, typically phosphatidylcholine (PC) that is a type of is a major component of cell membranes and a source of the essential nutrient choline.

Phosphatidylcholine is found in foods such as eggs, soybeans, and sunflower seeds and is crucial for maintaining the structure and function of cell membranes. It is also involved in synthesizing acetylcholine, a neurotransmitter important for memory and other functions.

Phytosomes are formed by chemically binding the hydrophilic (water-fearing) parts of phospholipids, such as phosphatidylcholine, to the plant-derived compounds.

The term "phyto" stands for plant, while "some" means cell-like. Phytosome is a technology for producing lipid-compatible (fat-soluble) drugs and nutraceutical standardized plant extracts to improve their absorption and bioavailability.

The novelty of the phytosome process lies in the fact that it produces a little cell, thus protecting the supplement from destruction by digestive enzymes and gut bacteria.

This creates a complex that has both water-loving (hydrophilic) and fat-loving (lipophilic) properties.

Phytosomes result in increased absorption and enhanced bioavailability of plant extracts by allowing them to pass more easily through the cell membranes, such as the gastrointestinal tract, so that the active plant compound reaches the bloodstream and target tissues.

CHAPTER TWENTY

Enhancing Cancer Immunotherapy with Vital Micronutrients (Vitamins and Minerals)

"A large body of evidence suggests that a significant percentage of deaths resulting from cancer could be avoided through greater attention to proper and adequate nutrition."

World J Clin Oncol

Raymond C-F Yuen [1], Shiu-Ying Tsao

2021 Sep 24;12(9):712–724. doi: 10.5306/wjco.v12.i9.712

https://pmc.ncbi.nlm.nih.gov/articles/PMC8479349/

Recent studies have suggested that nutrients available in the Tumor Micro Environment can positively influence immunotherapy response and cancer cell metabolic pathways.

"Micronutrients, in combination with checkpoint inhibitors, may enhance immunotherapy efficacy by immunomodulation (stimulating the immune response) and minimizing immune-related adverse events (side effects), improve acquired immune response through modification of the tumor microenvironment, enhance gut-microbiota immune functions, boost immune-nutrition function, and improve patient outcome.

Micronutrients such as vitamins A, beta-carotene, B2 (riboflavin), B6 (pyridoxine), B9 (folate), B12 (cobalamin), and benfotiamine (fat-soluble B12), C, D, E, Zinc, iron, copper, and selenium are excellent immune stimulators.

According to some studies, micronutrients with the strongest evidence for immune support are vitamin C, vitamin D, zinc, and selenium, which may all have immunomodulating functions to enhance the immune response rates of immunotherapy and even reduce irAE (Immune Response Adverse Effects).

These micronutrients play an important role in reducing oxidative stress in diseases and cancers.

Vitamin A supplementation improves levels of IgA immunoglobulin and CD40 ligand-activated IgG and reduces inflammatory cytokine levels.

Vitamin E is a potent antioxidant that can reduce inflammation by modulating T cell function and downmodulating prostaglandin E2 (works with specific receptors on cancer cells to augment healing).

Vitamin C. In higher doses, Vitamin C can influence PD-L1 expression through various pathways. It also improves immune functions by supporting natural killer cell activities, lymphocyte proliferation, and chemotaxis, stimulates dendritic cells to secrete interleukin-12, and activates T and B cell functions. High-dose vitamin C enhances the cytotoxic activity of CD8 T cells.

Vitamin C enhances immunotherapy by cooperating with immune checkpoint-inhibiting therapy.

It also reduces the formation of neutrophil extracellular traps in the Tumor Micro Environment, which are related to irAEs (immune-related adverse Events). The combination of high-dose vitamin C and immune checkpoint therapy may enhance the efficacy of immunotherapy for cancer.

Vitamin B12 deficiency has been linked to low lymphocyte counts, impaired NK cell function, decreased CD8+ cells, and impaired immune functions. Eventually, the raised CD4/CD8 ratio would be potentially reversible by oral or intramuscular B12 injections. Vitamin B12 supplements may reduce the side effects of immunotherapy because it is required for red blood cell synthesis, neural functions, and the reduction of the severity of drug-induced peripheral neuropathy.

Vitamin D binds to the vitamin D receptor of both the antigen-presenting cells (APC), dendritic cells, and T lymphocytes, which is a change towards a more tolerogenic (capable of producing immunological tolerance) state with induction of T helper-2 (Th2) lymphocytes and regulatory T lymphocytes (Tregs).

Vitamin D also inhibits inflammatory cytokine production by monocytes and suppresses dendritic cell differentiation and maturation. This helps to maintain tolerance and promotes protective immunity.

Studies have also shown that Vitamin D supplementation suppresses tumor angiogenesis (the blood vessels that feed cancer cells) and metastasis by targeting the Tumor Microenvironment.

The active form of vitamin D regulates stromal cells, including tumor-associated fibroblasts, tumor-derived endothelial cells, cancer stem cells, and infiltrating immune cells within the TME to facilitate cancer suppression. The anti-inflammatory effects of Vitamin D within the TME lead to the inhibition of cancer cell proliferation, induction of apoptosis, and autophagic cell death of cancer tumor cells.

Moreover, vitamin D supplementation has been shown to significantly increase gut microbial diversity.

A cohort study from the Mayo Clinic has shown a 26% reduction in non-small cell lung cancer mortality with improved quality of life and prolonged survival through micronutrients.

It may be applied with immunotherapy to improve immune functions, modulate the acquired immune response, decrease treatment toxicity, and enhance patient outcomes. Micronutrients such as selenium, vitamin C, and vitamin D (at high doses) are effective and safe for patients undergoing cancer treatment.

A recent cohort study has shown that vitamin D supplementation could reduce the risks of CPI-induced colitis by as much as 65%, as well as other CPI-induced and autoimmune-related irAEs.

Zinc

Zinc is an essential trace mineral. A typical dose is 15 mg/ day.

Research shows that zinc plays a role in modulating the expression and function of PD-1 on T-cells and immunity.

A zinc deficiency can result in impaired immune function. Zinc influences cell proliferation and programmed cell death. Zinc is an essential element that is integral to many proteins and transcription factors, which regulate key cellular functions such as the response to oxidative stress, DNA replication, DNA damage repair, cell cycle progression, and apoptosis.

Malignant cells exhibit significantly decreased zinc compared to normal cells. Two significant gene mutations are implicated in cancer. P53 and P21. P53, referred to as the "guardian of the genome," is a crucial tumor suppressor gene that plays a vital role in preventing cancer by regulating cell growth and death. P21 has functions such as regulating the cell cycle. Inhibiting cell proliferation and inducing apoptosis in cancer cells. With mutations, these genes do not function properly, and cancer can proliferate and tumors can grow.

Studies show that Zinc is crucial for the proper structure and function of the P53 protein, a vital tumor suppressor. The p53 protein's binding domain requires a zinc ion for correct functioning. Restoring zinc levels, particularly in cancer cells with mutated P53, can reactivate the protein and potentially inhibit tumor growth. In 1999, Liang *et al.* first reported that "zinc inhibits human prostatic carcinoma cell growth, possibly due to induction of cell cycle arrest and apoptosis."

Zinc appears to also directly influence P21, with zinc deficiency reducing its protective activity and zinc supplementation increasing it.

Selenium

Selenium, a trace element, plays a crucial role in immune function and has shown promise in enhancing immunotherapy outcomes in cancer treatment. Research suggests that selenium, particularly selenium nanoparticles, can boost the effectiveness of immunotherapy by enhancing immune cell activity and promoting anti-tumor immunity.

Selenium can enhance the toxicity of Natural Killer Cells and can improve the body's natural immune response to tumors, making immunotherapy more effective. The recommended dosage is 200 mcg a day, which can be found naturally in two Brazil nuts.

Proper nutrition maximizes the immune system to kill cancer.

CHAPTER TWENTY-ONE

Conclusion

A "cancer checkpoint" in immunotherapy refers to a protein on the surface of an immune cell, such as a T-Cell, that can act as an "immune cell off/on switch." These checkpoints are exploited by cancer cells to evade immune detection. Cancer cells can also express high levels of checkpoints, which trick the immune system into avoiding them. Immunotherapy's amazing success is based upon its ability to block these checkpoints with drugs called "checkpoint inhibitors," which are different types of monoclonal antibodies that cause the immune system to be reactivated to recognize, target, attack, destroy, and remember cancer cells.   Go to the following link for a Video Summary of Checkpoint Inhibitors:

https://video.search.yahoo.com/search/video?fr=mcafee&p=immunology+ch eckpoint+video&type=E211US1274G0#id=1&vid=a0622187ebb2d8bf05720ec 3c6bd43c9&action=click

Examples of "checkpoint" proteins include PD1 and CTLA-4 found on the surface of T-cells; and their ligand partners, PD-L1, and /B7-1, found on the surfaces of Cancer tumors. When the T-Cell and Tumor Cell checkpoint signals join, the immune system is turned off, and the cancer cells go rampant.

The checkpoint inhibitor's application of monoclonal antibodies that block checkpoint inhibitors and disrupt this signal is a type of immunotherapy that has had breakthrough curative effects.

Activating T-cells against cancer cells is the basis behind checkpoint inhibitors, which are a relatively new class of immunotherapy drugs that have recently been FDA-approved to treat lung cancer, metastatic melanoma, and more than 30 other cancers.

Targets for Different Checkpoint Inhibitors:

- anti-CTLA-4 therapies: ipilimumab (Yervoy) and tremelimumab (imjudo)

- anti-PD-1 therapies: cemiplimab, dostarlimab, nivolumab, pembrolizumab, retifanlimab-dlwr, and tislelizumab

- anti-PD-L1 therapies: atezolizumab, avelumab, and durvalumab

Name	Target	Approved

Name	Target	Approved
Nivolumab	PD-1	2014
Pembrolizumab	PD-1	2014
Atezolizumab	PD-L1	2016
Avelumab	PD-L1	2017
Durvalumab	PD-L1	2017
Cemiplimab	PD-1	2018
Tislelizumab	PD-1	2019
Dostarlimab	PD-1	2021
Retifanlimab	PD-1	2023
Toripalimab	PD-1	2023
Cosibelimab	PD-L1	2024

Types of Cancer Shown to Respond to Immunotherapy Checkpoint Inhibitors include, but are not limited to:

- Alveolar and part sarcoma
- B-Cell Lymphoma
- bile duct cancer
- bladder cancer
- breast cancer
- cervical cancer
- colorectal - colon cancer
- endometrial cancer
- esophageal cancer
- head and neck cancer
- Hodgkin lymphoma
- liver cancer
- lung cancer
- melanoma
- Merkel cell cancer
- mesothelioma
- ovarian cancer
- prostrate cancer
- rectal cancer
- renal cell cancer (kidney cancer)
- skin cancer
- stomach cancer
- soft tissue sarcomas

This is THE END...

OF CANCER!

www.ingramcontent.com/pod-product-compliance
Lightning Source LLC
Chambersburg PA
CBHW080420030426
42335CB00020B/2525